高职高专院校专业基础课纸数融合系列教材

供临床医学、口腔医学、护理、助产、药学、影像、检验等专业使用

# 高职医护英语

## GAOZHI YIHU YINGYU

主　编　江晓东　晏柳清　王　铭

副主编　冉凌云　殷沨君　吴丹迪　陈琰晗

编　者　（按姓氏笔画排序）

王　铭　重庆市中医院

冉凌云　昆明医科大学

刘东碧　重庆大学附属三峡医院

江晓东　重庆三峡医药高等专科学校

吴丹迪　重庆三峡医药高等专科学校

何晓磊　肇庆医学高等专科学校

张　莹　雅安职业技术学院

陈琰晗　重庆医科大学

晏柳清　重庆三峡医药高等专科学校

殷沨君　重庆三峡学院

唐科堉　四川护理职业学院

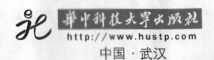

华中科技大学出版社

http://www.hustp.com

中国·武汉

## 内 容 简 介

本书为高职高专院校专业基础课纸数融合系列教材。

本书分为10个单元。每个单元以人体系统为主题,涉及提高学生相关信息收集能力的医学图表,提高学生医护职业场景会话能力的情景对话,以及提高学生浅显医护英语文章阅读能力的医学相关文章。

本书参考全国医护英语水平考试(METS)大纲的部分要求,针对职业院校医药专业学生的具体情况进行编写。本书体现"实用为主""够用为度"的思路,力图使教学内容与学生职业场景相结合。

本书可供医药类院校临床医学、药学、护理、医学技术等各专业学生学习,亦可供有初步英语基础的医护人员在职自主学习。

**图书在版编目(CIP)数据**

高职医护英语/江晓东,晏柳清,王铭主编.—武汉:华中科技大学出版社,2021.1(2022.8重印)
ISBN 978-7-5680-6824-6

Ⅰ.①高…　Ⅱ.①江…　②晏…　③王…　Ⅲ.①医学-英语-高等职业教育-教材　Ⅳ.①R

中国版本图书馆 CIP 数据核字(2021)第 012506 号

**高职医护英语**　　　　　　　　　　　　　　　　　江晓东　晏柳清　王　铭　主编
Gaozhi Yihu Yingyu

策划编辑:居　颖
责任编辑:曾奇峰　郭逸贤
封面设计:原色设计
责任校对:曾　�
责任监印:周治超

出版发行:华中科技大学出版社(中国·武汉)　　　电话:(027)81321913
　　　　　武汉市东湖新技术开发区华工科技园　　　邮编:430223
录　　排:华中科技大学惠友文印中心
印　　刷:武汉市籍缘印刷厂
开　　本:889mm×1194mm　1/16
印　　张:11.5
字　　数:　千字
版　　次:　年8月第1版第2次印刷
定　　价:　元

# 网络增值服务使用说明

欢迎使用华中科技大学出版社医学资源网yixue.hustp.com

## 1.教师使用流程

（1）登录网址：http://yixue.hustp.com （注册时请选择教师用户）

注册 ▶ 登录 ▶ 完善个人信息 ▶ 等待审核

（2）审核通过后，您可以在网站使用以下功能：

管理学生

建立课程　　　　　　　　　布置作业

下载教学资源　　　　教师　　　　查询学生学习记录等

## 2.学员使用流程

建议学员在PC端完成注册、登录、完善个人信息的操作。

（1）PC端学员操作步骤

①登录网址：http://yixue.hustp.com （注册时请选择普通用户）

注册 ▶ 登录 ▶ 完善个人信息

②查看课程资源

如有学习码，请在个人中心-学习码验证中先验证，再进行操作。

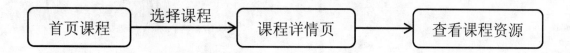

首页课程 —选择课程→ 课程详情页 → 查看课程资源

（2）手机端扫码操作步骤

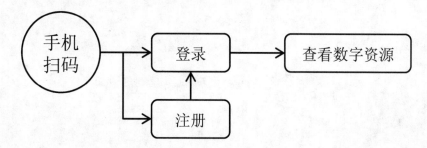

手机扫码 → 登录 → 查看数字资源

注册

# Preface | 前　言

为更新英语课堂教学的内容和方式,更好地为医护专业人才培养服务,我们组织有关教师和医护专业人员,根据《医护英语入门教程》在课堂教学中的使用反馈,对其进行了大量修改和补充,编写了本书。本书参考全国医护英语水平考试(METS)大纲的部分要求,针对职业院校医药专业学生的具体情况进行编写,旨在通过情景对话、专业阅读训练,培养医药专业学生在实际工作中综合应用英语的能力。

本书在编写过程中针对职业院校医药专业学生的英语基础学力和学习心理特点,以专门用途英语的相关理论为指导,将英语教学的新模式与医药科学的新知识、新进展、新观念有机整合,内容新颖、充实,注重实用性和时代性,强化以学生发展为本的理念,适应课堂任务型教学和注重学生自主学习能力的培养。

本书共 10 个单元。医学图表部分旨在提高学生学习兴趣和培养学生从医学图表中获取重要信息的能力。情景对话部分以医疗服务流程中常见情景为题材,学生可以根据这些对话,学会用英语准确流利地与患者或同事沟通。课文部分以医药领域新进展为主题,希望学生在英语阅读中积累医药核心词汇,同时了解医药领域的信息和资讯。部分文章以常见疾病为主题,涉及这些疾病的概念、症状、治疗、预防等,通过这些短文的阅读,学生能够熟悉和掌握高频医学词汇。课后练习含相关词汇练习、阅读理解练习和翻译练习。全书附录包括常见医用英语缩写词、对话部分文本、课文翻译、课后参考答案。

本书编写工作分工如下:第一单元、第四单元由江晓东编写;第二单元、第三单元由晏柳清编写;第五单元由何晓磊编写;第六单元由张莹编写;第七单元由殷沕君编写;第八单元由王铭编写;第九单元由吴丹迪编写;第十单元由陈琰晗编写;Midterm Review 和 Final Review 部分由唐科堉编写;各单元对话和附录 A 由冉凌云编写;附录 B 由刘东碧编写。

本书在课文选材时参阅了大量书籍、网页和报刊资料,对这些资料的作者和提供者表示衷心感谢。在编写过程中,重庆医药高等专科学校王炎峰老师、重庆三峡医药高等专科学校教师 Carolyn Kreuzkamp、Sara Wei 提供了大量文章素材和关于本书编写的宝贵建议,在此一并表示衷心感谢。

鉴于时间紧迫和编者能力有限,书中可能还存在错漏之处,敬请读者批评指正。缩略语仅供阅读英文专业材料时参考,非临床使用标准。特别提示:本书图片、对话、练习和课文所提供信息不能替代专业医护咨询或诊治。

编　者

# 目 录
MULU

# Unit 1　The Cardiovascular System

## Learning Objectives:

To remember some key English words related to the cardiovascular system.

To understand the conversation about receiving a patient and talk about the topic.

To read and understand the main ideas and the details of the passages about the cardiovascular system.

To learn to write a birthday certificate with the help of the given sample writing.

To learn by heart some word roots, prefixes and suffixes about the circulatory system.

## Part 1　Look and Learn

**Warming-up 1: Look at the following picture, talk about them and then finish Task 1.**

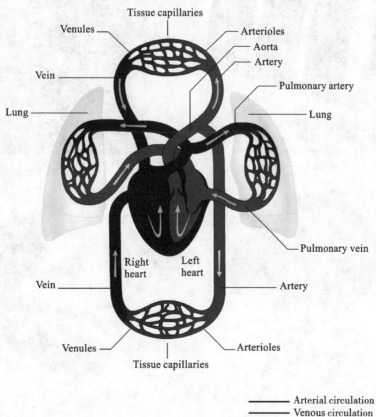

*Note*

## New Words

vein [veɪn] n. 静脉

artery [ˈɑːtərɪ] n. 动脉

capillary [kəˈpɪlərɪ] n. 毛细血管

tissue [ˈtɪʃuː] n. （人体）组织

pulmonary [ˈpʌlmənərɪ] adj. 肺部的

lung [lʌŋ] n. 肺

aorta [eɪˈɔːtə] n. 主动脉

arteriole [ɑːˈtɪərɪəʊl] n. 小动脉

**Task 1　Match the words in the left column with the explanations in the right column.**

| 1. heart | A. either of the two organs in the chest with which people and some animals breathe |
| --- | --- |
| 2. lung | B. the main artery |
| 3. aorta | C. a very thin tube that carry blood around the body |
| 4. capillary | D. a tube that carries blood to the heart from the other parts of the body |
| 5. vein | E. the organ in the chest that sends the blood around the body |

**Warming-up 2：Look at the following pictures about medical instruments，talk about them and then finish Task 2.**

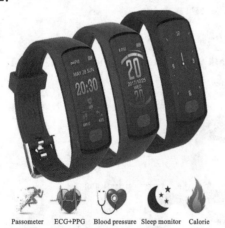

Passometer　ECG+PPG　Blood pressure　Sleep monitor　Calorie

(1)

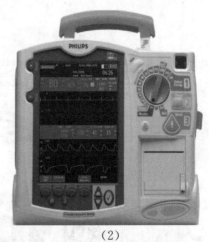

(2)

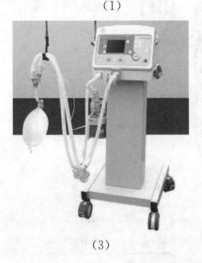

(3)

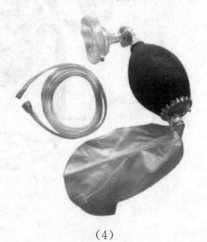

(4)

## New Words

bracelet ['breɪslɪt] n. 手环

monitor ['mɒnɪtə(r)] n. 监护仪

respirator ['respəreɪtə(r)] n. 呼吸机

**Task 2  Match the picture number with the proper English and Chinese meaning.**

| Picture number | English | Chinese |
|---|---|---|
|  | fitness bracelet | 运动手环 |
|  | ECG monitor | 心电监护仪 |
|  | simple respirator | 简易呼吸器 |
|  | respirator | 呼吸器 |

# Part 2   Listen and Learn

## Situation Dialogue：Receiving a Patient

**Task 3   Listen to the audio episode one and fill in the missing words referring to the original text. Then check your writing against the original.**

Doctor：Good morning. I am Doctor Sterling. How can I help you?

Patient：Good morning, Doctor. I am Emily. I have a 1. _____ and 2. _____ since yesterday.

Doctor：Oh, did you take your temperature?

Patient：Yes, I did. The highest temperature was 39.8 ℃ at 11:00 pm last night. I took one pill of aspirin and feel much better.

Doctor：Any other symptoms?

Patient：I have a 3. _____ and 4. _____, too.

Doctor：OK, let me take your temperature first. Please keep this thermometer under your armpit for 5 minutes. Open your mouth and say "Ah", please. Your tonsils and larynx are red and swollen. Your temperature is 38.5 ℃. Your breathing sounds are normal and there is no problem with your lungs. You'd better take the 5. _____, OK? This paper is for the lab test.

Patient：Sure. I really hope I get better as soon as possible. See you later.

扫码听
对话1

**Task 4   Listen to the audio episode two and complete the answers according to the questions.**

1. What does the result of blood test indicate?

   The result indicates that the patient has an _____ respiratory tract infection.

2. If fever persists, what should the patient do?

   The patient should _____ if fever persists.

3. How should the patient take the medicine?

   The patient should take it _____ a day.

扫码听
对话2

*Note*

扫码听
课文 A

# Part 3　Read and Learn

**Passage A**

## The Cardiovascular System and Related Disease in China

**The heart and circulatory system**

The heart and circulatory system (also called the cardiovascular system) make up the network that delivers blood to the body's tissues. With each heartbeat, blood is sent throughout our bodies, carrying oxygen and nutrients to all of our cells.

Every day, the approximately 10 pints (5 liters) of blood in the body travel many times through about 60,000 miles (96,560 kilometers) of blood vessels that branch and cross, linking the cells of our organs and body parts. From the hard-working heart, to the thickest arteries, to capillaries so thin that they can only be seen through a microscope, the cardiovascular system is our body's lifeline.

The circulatory system is composed of the heart and blood vessels, including arteries, veins, and capillaries. Our bodies actually have two circulatory systems: the pulmonary circulation is a short loop from the heart to the lungs and back again, and the systemic circulation (the system we usually think of as our circulatory system) sends blood from the heart to all the other parts of our bodies and back again.

**Cardiovascular disease (CVD) in China**

A rise in cardiovascular disease (CVD) in China appears to have been spurred largely by increases in high blood pressure. Increasing body mass index (BMI), decreasing physical activity, a high prevalence of smoking, and unhealthy diet have also contributed to the growing burden of CVD, which now is the leading cause of death in China.

A wide range of dietary, lifestyle, and metabolic risk factors may be impacting CVD burden in China. The major changes in Chinese society, including a dramatic shift from a traditional to a more "Western" diet and lifestyle and rapid urbanization and industrialization, may have contributed to the jump in cardiovascular diseases, such as heart attack and stroke. These changes have been accompanied by marked increases in high cholesterol, obesity, and type Ⅱ diabetes among the Chinese population. Prevention of these diseases through promoting healthy diet and lifestyle should be increased to a national public policy priority.

## New Words

circulatory [ˌsɜːkjʊˈleɪtərɪ] adj. 循环的

cardiovascular [ˌkɑːdɪəʊˈvæskjʊlə(r)] adj. 心血管的

nutrient [ˈnjuːtrɪənt] n. 营养物

approximately [əˈprɒksɪmətlɪ] adv. 大约

systemic [sɪˈstemɪk] adj. 全身的,系统的

prevalence [ˈprevələns] n. 发病率

metabolic [ˌmetəˈbɒlɪk] adj. 代谢的

stroke [strəʊk] n. 脑卒中

cholesterol [kəˈlestərɒl] n. 胆固醇

obesity [əʊˈbiːsətɪ] n. 肥胖

*Note*

**Task 5　Fill in the blanks with the words given below and change the word forms if necessary.**

1. The blood _____(circulatory) is maintained by the heart, which consists of two pumps that feed separate circuits.

2. The expectant mothers can attend the classes and learn about having a healthy pregnancy and _____(deliver).

3. The dietitian is explaining to the patient that some of the diseases may be prevented by improving _____(nutrient).

4. An _____(approximately) number is a nearly correct but not exact one.

5. The paper introduces _____(systematic) the function and structure of human beings' hearts.

6. The _____(prevalent) rate of this disease was investigated in that region.

7. The physically inactive patient had an _____(health) diet and he did no exercises.

8. _____(urbanize) began during the Industrial Revolution, when worker moved towards cities.

9. Chongqing is the commercial and _____(industrialization) center in Southwest China.

10. The science of medicine is traditionally classified in basic medicine, _____ (prevention) medicine, clinical medicine and rehabilitation medicine.

**Task 6　Choose the correct answer according to the passage.**

1. What is the main function of the heart and circulatory system? _____

A. It produces oxygen and nutrients to the cells of our bodies

B. It helps people inhale and exhale oxygen for the internal organs of the body

C. It sends blood all over the body and transports oxygen and nutrients to the cells

D. It is used to help pregnant women deliver babies

2. Which of the followings is a larger measurement unit for volume? _____

A. pint　　　　　B. liter　　　　　C. mile　　　　　D. kilometer

3. What is connecting the cells of our organs and body parts? _____

A. heart　　　　　B. lung　　　　　C. blood vessels　　　D. veins

4. Which of the following statements is true according to the passage? _____

A. Arteries and capillaries are so thin that they can only be seen through a microscope

B. The cardiovascular system is vital to our bodies

C. The circulatory system is composed of arteries and veins

D. The pulmonary circulation is a short loop from the heart to the lungs and to all the other parts of our bodies and back again

5. Which is mentioned in this passage as a contributing factor to the rise of cardiovascular disease in China? _____

A. the addiction to the use of electronic products like smart phones

B. the overuse, misuse and abuse of antibiotics

C. the trend in urbanization, globalization and industrialization

D. the physically inactive lifestyle

**Task 7　Arrange the following steps about cardiopulmonary resuscitation in proper sequence based on the medical procedure.**

_____ Continue CPR: Complete 15 compressions, give two effective breaths (EAR), and

*Note*

5

continue compressions and breaths in ratio of 15 : 2 at a rate of 4 cycles per minute. Check pulse about every minute.

_____ Keep thumb of one hand in position and place heel of the other hand below it, place heel of the other hand on top of first and interlock fingers of both hands.

_____ Commence chest compressions: Position yourself vertically above casualty's chest, with your arms strait, press down on breastbone to depress it about 4-5 cm, release pressure.

_____ Position hands for CPR: Place casualty on back, find groove at neck between collarbones, find lower end of breastbone by running, finger along last rib to centre of body, extend thumbs equal distances to meet in middle of breastbone.

## New Words

resuscitation [rɪˌsʌsɪ'teɪʃən] n. 恢复知觉,苏醒
ratio ['reɪʃɪəʊ] n. 比,比率
vertically ['vɜːtɪkəlɪ] adv. 垂直地,直立地
casualty ['kæʒjʊəltɪ] n. 受害者,死伤者

扫码听
课文B

**Passage B**

### Hypertension

High blood pressure, termed "hypertension", is a condition that afflicts almost 1 billion people worldwide and is a leading cause of morbidity and mortality. Many people are not even aware that they are hypertensive. Therefore, this disease is sometimes called the "silent killer". This disease is usually asymptomatic until the damaging effects of hypertension (such as stroke, myocardial infarction, renal dysfunction and visual problems) are observed.

Hypertension is defined as an abnormal elevation of blood pressure. Both systolic and diastolic pressure values are important to note. According to some U. S. national diagnosis guidelines, the following values represent different stages of hypertension.

| Classification | Systolic pressure/mmHg | Diastolic pressure/mmHg |
|---|---|---|
| Normal | <120 | <80 |
| Prehypertension | 120-139 | 80-89 |
| Stage 1 | 140-160 | 90-100 |
| Stage 2 | >160 | >100 |

In 90%-95% of patients presenting with hypertension, the cause is unknown. This condition is called primary (or essential) hypertension. The remaining 5%-10% of hypertensive patients have hypertension that results secondarily from renal disease, endocrine disorders, or other identifiable causes. This form of hypertension is called secondary hypertension.

A hypertensive crisis is a severe increase in blood pressure that can lead to a stroke. Extremely high blood pressure, above 180/110 millimeters of mercury (mmHg), damages blood vessels. The heart may not be able to maintain adequate circulation of blood. A hypertensive crisis is divided into two categories: urgent and emergency. Signs and symptoms of an urgent hypertensive crisis may include elevated blood pressure, severe headache, severe anxiety, and shortness of breath. During an emergency hypertensive crisis, you may experience life-threatening signs and symptoms, such as pulmonary edema, brain swelling or bleeding, heart attack and stroke.

In most cases of hypertension, doctors can't point to the exact cause. But several things are known to raise blood pressure, including being very overweight, drinking too much alcohol, having a family history of high blood pressure, eating too much salt, and getting older. Your blood pressure may also rise if you are not very active or you don't eat enough potassium and calcium.

High blood pressure doesn't usually cause symptoms. Most people don't know that they have it until they go to the doctor for some other reasons. Without treatment, high blood pressure can damage the heart, brain, kidneys, or eyes. This damage causes problems like coronary artery disease, stroke, and kidney failure. Very high blood pressure can cause headaches, vision problems, nausea, and vomiting.

Treatment depends on how high your blood pressure is, whether you have other health problems such as diabetes, and whether any organs have already been damaged. Your doctor will also consider how likely you are to develop other diseases, especially heart disease. Most people with hypertension are treated with antihypertensive medications. Hypertension is also commonly treated with drugs that decrease cardiac output. Vasodilator drugs, which decrease systemic vascular resistance, are also used to treat hypertension.

You can help lower your blood pressure by making healthy changes in your lifestyle. If those lifestyle changes don't work, you may also need to take pills. Lifestyle changes you can make to help prevent high blood pressure are as follows.

· Lose extra weight.

· Eat less salt.

· Exercise.

· Limit alcohol.

· Get 3,500 mg of potassium in your diet every day. Fresh, unprocessed whole foods have the most potassium. These foods include meat, fish, nonfat and low-fat dairy products, and many fruits and vegetables.

## New Words

afflict [əˈflɪkt] vt. 使痛苦，折磨

antihypertensive [ˈæntɪˌhaɪpəˈtensɪv] adj. & n. 抗高血压的（药物）

asymptomatic [ˌeɪsɪmptəˈmætɪk] adj. 无症状的

calcium [ˈkælsɪəm] n. 钙

cardiac [ˈkɑːdɪæk] n. 强心剂
　　　　　　　　　adj. 心脏的

diastolic [ˌdaɪəˈstɒlɪk] adj. 心脏舒张的

dysfunction [dɪsˈfʌŋkʃən] n. 功能紊乱，功能障碍

hypertension [ˌhaɪpəˈtenʃən] n. 高血压

mercury [ˈmɜːkjʊrɪ] n. 水银，汞

mortality [mɔːˈtælətɪ] n. 死亡率

potassium [pəʊˈtæsɪəm] n. 钾

secondary [ˈsekəndərɪ] adj. 次要的，二级的

stroke [strəʊk] n. 打击，脑卒中

systolic [ˌsɪsˈtɒlɪk] adj. 心脏收缩的

unprocessed [ˌʌnˈprəʊsest] adj. 未被加工的

vascular [ˈvæskjʊlə(r)] adj. 脉管的，血管的

vasodilator [ˌveɪzəʊdaɪˈleɪtə(r)] adj. 血管扩张的
　　　　　　　　　n. 血管扩张剂

*Note*

## Exercises

**Task 8   Match the words or phrases with similar meaning in the two columns.**

| A | B |
|---|---|
| 1. hypertension | a. additional |
| 2. approximately | b. obstruct |
| 3. vision | c. raise |
| 4. systemic | d. trouble |
| 5. elevate | e. fatty deposits |
| 6. category | f. about |
| 7. afflict | g. high blood pressure |
| 8. block | h. sight |
| 9. atheroma | i. all over the body |
| 10. extra | j. kind |

**Task 9   Choose the right answer to fill in the blanks in the passage.**

In the hospital's __1__ area, a little girl cried as the doctors __2__ a foot torn open. A boy, 11, quietly passed away on his hospital __3__ , and his father wept. A nurse pushed through the crowd and blood splattered across her white __4__ and headscarf. This is an average day at this hospital in central Aleppo. Every day, 70 to 100 __5__ pass through the doors here, 80 percent of which are civilians. Most patients arrive here on the back of pick-up trucks. Of the hospital's five __6__ , only one remains. The lone ambulance driver, Sam, who before was a wedding dress designer, said: "Before I designed only for women. Now I work for all humanity." When an __7__ rocked the street outside the hospital, civilians ran for cover. Several doctors raced toward the sound of the blast to look for __8__ . Sam rushed to his van. "My family has to flee the city. But I can't leave my post." said one of the nurses. Like many of the doctors, none of these women had prior experience in __9__ . But now they are practically experts in the __10__ of trauma patients.

1. A. reception    B. receive    C. belief    D. believe
2. A. saved    B. stitched    C. cured    D. steamed
3. A. chair    B. sofa    C. bed    D. furniture
4. A. reform    B. inform    C. formation    D. uniform
5. A. patients    B. doctors    C. nurses    D. directors
6. A. trucks    B. ambulances    C. buses    D. taxis
7. A. explode    B. explosive    C. explosion    D. exploration
8. A. survive    B. surviving    C. survival    D. survivors
9. A. medicine    B. teaching    C. cooking    D. singing
10. A. treat    B. treatment    C. move    D. movement

## Part 4   Write and Learn

**Birth Certificate**

**Direction: Read the following writing sample carefully. Design and finish an imitated writing task**

**with similar style.**

出生证明

出生证明是一份重要文件,它包括以下内容:婴儿的性别、出生时间、出生地点,父母的姓名,婴儿的身高,婴儿的体重。

【Sample】

Birth Certificate

This is to certify that Wang Ming (male) was born on March 18th, 2008 in Shenyang, China, to Wang Dashang, father, and Li Yan, mother. Weight:3.6 kg. Length:51 cm.

The People's Hospital of Shenyang

(sealed)

Signature:

(sealed)

April 23rd, 2008

【Assignment】

Write a birth certificate according to the following information.

姓名:刘阳 性别:女 体重:3.1 kg 身高:48 cm

出生日期:2008 年 5 月 1 日

出生地:上海市第一人民医院

父亲姓名:刘宏伟 母亲姓名:江丽红

# Part 5 Prefixes, Suffixes & Roots

Circulatory System (循环系统)

| 汉语(英语) | 常用词根 | 例 词 |
|---|---|---|
| 心(heart) | cardi(o)-; -cardium | electrocardiogram 心电图;carditis 心肌炎; phonocardiogram 心音图;cardiology 心脏病学;myocardium 心肌层; pericardium 心包膜 |
| 心房(atrium) | atri(o)- | atriotomy 心房切开术;periatrial 心房周的;transatrial 经心房的;atrial 心房的 |
| 心室(ventricle) | ventricul- | supraventricular 室上的;ventriculocentesis 心室穿刺术; ventriculofiberscopy 心室纤维镜检查 |
| 瓣膜(valve) | valvul(o)- | valvulitis 瓣膜炎;multivalvular 多瓣膜的;valvulopathy 心瓣膜病 |
| 血管(vessel) | vas(o)-; angi(o)- | vasculitis 血管炎;vasopressin 血管升压素;angiotensin 血管紧张素; angiography 血管造影 |
| 动脉(artery) | arteri(o)- | arteriography 动脉造影术;arteritis 动脉炎;endoarteritis 动脉内膜炎; arteriosclerosis 动脉硬化 |
| 静脉(vein) | ven(o)-; phleb(o)- | venous 静脉的;intravenous 内静脉的;phlebitis 静脉炎;phlebography 静脉造影 |
| 脉搏(pulse) | puls(o)- | pulseless 无脉的;pulsed 脉冲的 |

**Task 10   Learn the prefixes, suffixes or roots in the table by heart and then choose the best answer to finish the exercises.**

1. The Chinese meaning for the word "angiotensin" is _____.

   A. 血管紧张素原       B. 血管成形       C. 血管舒缩活动       D. 血管紧张素

2. The correct spelling form for "静脉造影" is _____ -graphy?

   A. veino       B. arter       C. vaso       D. phlebo

3. What's the combining form for the medical term "心音图" :phono- _____ -gram?

   A. heart       B. cardi       C. cardio       D. cor

4. The Chinese explanation for "endoarteritis" is _____.

   A. 动脉炎       B. 脉管炎       C. 动脉内膜炎       D. 主动脉炎

5. The English term for "静脉炎" is _____.

   A. phlebitis       B. veinitis       C. venitis       D. venulitis

6. The word combining "arterio" with "graphy" means _____.

   A. 动脉成形术       B. 动脉造影术       C. 动脉石       D. 动脉内膜炎

7. To make a word pertaining to the heart and blood vessels is _____.

   A. cardioventricular   B. cardioversion       C. cardiovalvular   D. cardiovascular

8. Which word in the following means inflammation of artery? _____

   A. arteritis       B. atritis       C. arthritis       D. angitis

9. The English equivalent for the word "血管炎" is _____.

   A. phlebitis                       B. vessel inflammation

   C. vasculitis                      D. angitis

10. Which form in the following has nothing to do with "脉搏"? _____

   A. pulse       B. impulse       C. pulso-       D. sphygmo-

# Unit 2    The Digestive System

## Learning Objectives:

To remember some key English words related to the digestive system.

To understand the conversation about consulting a doctor and talk about the topic.

To read and understand the main ideas and the details of the passages about the digestive system.

To learn to write a doctor's certificate with the help of the given sample writing.

To learn by heart some word roots, prefixes and suffixes about the digestive system.

## Part 1    Look and Learn

**Warming-up 1: Look at the following picture, talk about them and then finish Task 1.**

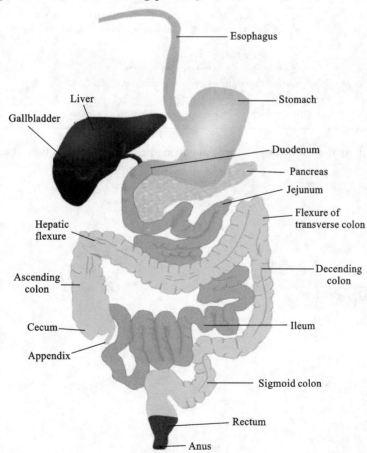

*Note*

## New Words

esophagus [iːˈsɒfəgəs] n. 食管

liver [ˈlɪvə(r)] n. 肝脏,(食用)肝

hepatic [hɪˈpætɪk] adj. 肝脏的,治肝病的,肝脏色的

gallbladder [ˈɡɔːlˌblædə(r)] n. 胆囊

duodenum [ˌdjuːəʊˈdiːnəm] n. 十二指肠

pancreas [ˈpæŋkrɪəs] n. 胰,胰腺

jejunum [dʒɪˈdʒuːnəm] n. 空肠

flexure [ˈflekʃə(r)] n. 屈曲,弯曲部分,打褶,挠曲

colon [ˈkəʊlən] n. 结肠

cecum [ˈsiːkəm] n. 盲肠

ileum [ˈɪlɪəm] n. 回肠

appendix [əˈpendɪks] n. 阑尾

rectum [ˈrektəm] n. 直肠

anus [ˈeɪnəs] n. 肛门

**Task 1　Match the words in the left column with the explanations in the right column.**

| 1. gallbladder | A. the first part of the small intestine immediately beyond the stomach |
|---|---|
| 2. colon | B. a muscular sac attached to the liver that stores bile secreted by the liver until it is needed for digestion |
| 3. duodenum | C. a large gland behind the stomach which produces digestive enzymes and releases them into the duodenum |
| 4. esophagus | D. the part of the large intestine between the cecum and the rectum |
| 5. pancreas | E. the muscular tube which connects the throat to the stomach |

　　**Warming-up 2：Look at the following pictures about medical instruments, talk about them and then finish Task 2.**

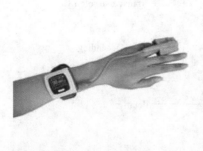
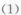

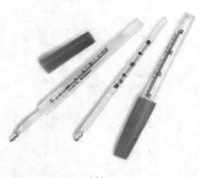

(1)　　　　　　　　　　　　　　　　(2)

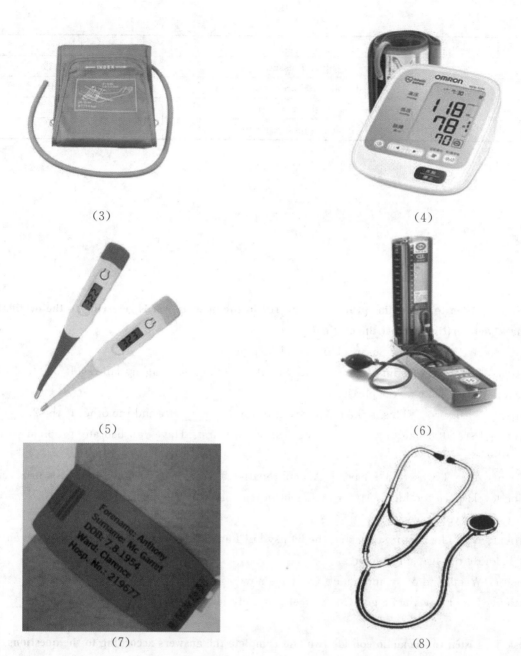

(3)

(4)

(5)

(6)

(7)

(8)

## New Words

monitor ['mɒnɪtə(r)] n. 显示屏，屏幕
thermometer [θə'mɒmɪtə(r)] n. 温度计，体温表
oximeter [ɒk'sɪmɪtə(r)] n. 血氧（定量）计
stethoscope ['steθəskəʊp] n. 听诊器

**Task 2  Match the picture number with the proper English and Chinese meaning.**

| Picture number | English | Chinese |
| --- | --- | --- |
|  | electric thermometer | 电子体温计 |
|  | stethoscope | 听诊器 |
|  | pulse oximeter | 脉搏血氧仪 |
|  | ID bracelet | 身份识别腕带 |

Note

续表

| Picture number | English | Chinese |
|---|---|---|
| | blood pressure cuff | 血压袖带 |
| | digital blood pressure monitor | 数字血压计 |
| | thermometer | 体温计 |
| | blood pressure monitor | 血压计 |

# Part 2   Listen and Learn

## Situation Dialogue：Consulting a Doctor

扫码听
对话 1

**Task 3   Listen to the audio episode one and fill in the missing words referring to the original text. Then check your writing against the original.**

Doctor：Hi，I am doctor Susan. How can I help you?

Patient：Hi，doctor. I am Mary. Would you please take a look at my lab result?

Doctor：Sure. Take a seat please.

Patient：Thank you. This is the blood result of my 1. _____ ，and the other is the 2. _____.

Doctor：I see. I'd like to know your medical history first. Have you had any problem with your kidney or liver?

Patient：Yes. I was told I have IgA nephropathy 5 years ago because both my uric acid and creatinine levels were too high. My urine has been tea-colored for almost 5 years.

Doctor：Did you have a 3. _____?

Patient：No. The doctor suggested the biopsy but I am really afraid of that. So they haven't been able to diagnose the IgA until now.

Doctor：What kind of symptoms do you have now?

Patient：Oh，I have had a gout for a week，and my left foot is still 4. _____ and 5. _____.

**Task 4   Listen to the audio episode two and complete the answers according to the questions.**

1. What is the patient taking for gout these days?

   The patient is taking a _____.

2. Why the patient should avoid the painkillers?

   Because the painkillers affect _____.

3. What's the doctor's suggestion?

   The doctor suggests trying some _____.

扫码听
对话 2

# Part 3   Read and Learn

**Passage A**

**Introduction to the Digestive System**

Every morsel of food we eat has to be broken down into nutrients that can be absorbed by the

Note

body, which is why it takes hours to fully digest food. In human beings, proteins must be broken down into amino acids, starches into simple sugars, and fats into fatty acids and glycerol. The water in our food and drink is also absorbed into the bloodstream to provide the body with the fluid which it needs.

The digestive system is made up of the alimentary canal and the other abdominal organs that play roles in digestion, such as the liver and the pancreas. The alimentary canal (also called the digestive tract) is a long tube of organs, including the esophagus, the stomach, and the intestines, that runs from the mouth to the anus. An adult's digestive tract is about 30 feet (9.144 meters) long.

The process of digestion starts well before food reaches the stomach. When we see, smell, taste, or even imagine a tasty snack, our salivary glands, which are located under the tongue and near the lower jaw, begin producing saliva. This flow of saliva is set in motion by a brain reflex that's triggered when we sense food or even think about eating. In response to this sensory stimulation, the brain sends impulses through the nerves that control the salivary glands, telling them to prepare for a meal.

During the process of absorption, nutrients that come from the food (including carbohydrates, proteins, fats, vitamins, and minerals) pass through channels in the intestinal wall and into the bloodstream. The blood works to distribute these nutrients to the rest of the body. The waste parts of food that the body can't use are passed out of the body as feces.

## New Words & Phrases

morsel ['mɔːsəl] n. 一口,(尤指食物)小块,碎屑

absorb [əb'sɔːb] v. 吸收,理解,掌握

digest [dɪ'dʒest] v. 消化,理解

protein ['prəʊtiːn] n. 朊,蛋白(质)

amino acid 氨基酸

glycerol ['glɪsərɒl] n. 甘油,丙三醇

alimentary [ˌælɪ'mentərɪ] adj. 食物的,营养的

alimentary canal 消化道

saliva [sə'laɪvə] n. 唾液,吐沫,涎

salivary gland 唾腺

carbohydrate [ˌkɑːbəʊ'haɪdreɪt] n. 碳水化合物,糖类,淀粉质或糖类食物

**Task 5   Fill in the blanks with the words given below and change the word forms if necessary.**

1. I convert the crisp fat in Joe's breakfast bacon into fatty acids and _____ (glycerol).

2. This breakdown process proceeds with the assistance of _____ (digest) enzymes secreted by the animals.

3. It continues with congenital and acquired _____ (salivary) dysfunction, including the goals for restoration of gland function.

4. Carbon, hydrogen and oxygen combine chemically to form _____ (carbohydrate) and fats.

5. The control of _____ (pancreas) secretion is performed mainly through two hormones.

6. Insects are made up of tens of thousands of _____ (protein).

7. Evidently, _____ (esophagus) cancer is a common disease in the elderly.

8. This diagnosis was confirmed by computed tomographic scan of the _____

*Note*

15

(abdominal).

9. To become transparent, an animal needs to keep its body from _____ (absorb) or scattering light.

10. Crude fatty materials contain certain substances that are not hydrolyzed in the human _____ (aliment) system.

**Task 6  Choose the correct answer according to the passage.**

1. Why does it take hours to fully digest food? _____

A. Because we eat a lot of food

B. Because we eat very little food

C. Because the food we eat is too hard

D. Because the food we eat has to be broken down into nutrients that can be absorbed by the body

2. Which of the following organs does not belong to the digestive system? _____

A. alimentary canal　　B. liver　　　　　C. pancreas　　　　　D. lung

3. When does the process of digestion start well? _____

A. before the food reaches the stomach

B. after the food reaches the stomach

C. as soon as the food reaches the stomach

D. all of the above

4. Where do the nutrients from the food pass through and into the bloodstream? _____

A. channels in the pancreatic wall

B. channels in the gastric wall

C. channels in the intestinal wall

D. channels in the hepatic wall

5. Which of the following statements is true according to the passage? _____

A. The water in our food and drink is also absorbed into the bloodstream to provide the body with the energy which it needs

B. The waste parts of food that the body can't use are passed out of the body as stools

C. The digestive tract is composed of esophagus, stomach and intestine

D. When we eat food, our salivary glands begin producing saliva

**Task 7  Arrange the following statements about digestive process in proper sequence based on the passage.**

_____ We eat different kinds of food.

_____ The waste parts of food that the body can't use are passed out of the body as feces.

_____ In the process of absorption, nutrients that come from the food pass through channels in the intestinal wall and into the bloodstream.

_____ Our salivary glands, which are located under the tongue and near the lower jaw, begin producing saliva.

**Passage B**

### Constipation

Constipation is a common digestive system problem in which you have infrequent bowel movements, pass hard stools, or strain during bowel movements. There may not be defecation for more than a few days.

Not having a bowel movement every day doesn't necessarily mean you're constipated. You're likely constipated, however, if you pass a hard stool fewer than three times a week, strain frequently during bowel movements, or have abdominal bloating or discomfort.

To understand constipation, it helps to know how the colon, or large intestine, works. As food moves through the colon, the colon absorbs water from the food while it forms waste products, or stools. Muscle contractions in the colon then push the stools toward the rectum. By the time stools reach the rectum, they are solids, because most of the water has been absorbed.

Constipation occurs when the colon absorbs too much water or if the colon muscle contractions are slow or sluggish, causing the stools to move through the colon too slowly. As a result, stools can become hard and dry. Common causes of constipation are as follows.

- Inadequate fluid intake.
- A low-fiber diet.
- Inattention to bowel habits.
- Age.
- Lack of physical activity.
- Pregnancy.
- Illness.

When you are constipated, you feel that passing stools has become more difficult than it used to be. Passing stools may be more difficult for one, or more reasons. For example, passing stools may have become significantly less frequent, or significantly less effective (you feel that you are unable to completely empty your bowel).

Most people do not need to worry extraordinarily. Only a small number of patients with constipation have more serious medical problems. If you have constipation for more than two weeks, you should see a doctor so that he or she can determine the source of your problem and treat it. If constipation is caused by colon cancer, early detection and treatment is very important.

A diagnosis of constipation generally depends on your medical history and physical exam. Your doctor will first want to make sure you don't have a blockage in your small intestine or colon (intestinal obstruction), an endocrine condition, such as hypothyroidism, or an electrolyte disturbance. He or she will also want to check your medications in case that they may be causing your constipation.

In people without medical problems, the main intervention is to increase the intake of fluids (preferably water) and dietary fiber. The latter may be achieved by consuming more vegetables, fruits and whole meal breads, and by adding linseed oil to one's diet. The routine non-medical use of laxatives is to be discouraged as this may result in bowel action becoming dependent upon their use. Enemas can be used to provide a form of mechanical stimulation. However, enemas are generally useful only for stools in the rectum, not in the intestinal tract.

## New Words

bowel ['baʊəl] n. 肠
constipation [ˌkɒnstɪ'peɪʃən] n. 便秘
consume [kən'sjuːm] vt. 消耗，消费，吸引
　　　　　　　vi. 消灭，毁灭
contraction [kən'trækʃən] n. 收缩，紧缩，(肌肉)痉挛
defecation [ˌdefɪ'keɪʃən] n. 澄清，净化，通便

electrolyte [ɪˈlektrəʊlaɪt] n. 电解质,电解液

enema [ˈenɪmə] n. 灌肠剂

hypothyroidism [ˌhaɪpəʊˈθaɪrɔɪdɪzəm] n. [医]甲状腺功能减退

intestinal [ɪnˈtestɪnəl] adj. 肠的,肠内的,(疾病)侵袭肠的

laxative [ˈlæksətɪv] adj. 放松的,通便的

linseed [ˈlɪnˌsiːd] n. 亚麻籽,亚麻仁

pregnancy [ˈpregnənsɪ] n. 怀孕

stimulation [ˌstɪmjʊˈleɪʃən] n. 激励,鼓舞,刺激

stool [stuːl] n. 大便

## Exercises

**Task 8   Match the words or phrases with similar meaning in the two columns.**

| A | B |
|---|---|
| 1. pregnancy | a. an underactive thyroid gland |
| 2. bowel | b. the part of intestine |
| 3. constipation | c. bowel movement |
| 4. defecation | d. inflammation of appendix |
| 5. contraction | e. any of the hormone-producing organs |
| 6. intestinal | f. with child |
| 7. endocrine | g. inability to regularly empty the bowels |
| 8. colon | h. intestine |
| 9. appendicitis | i. muscle spasm |
| 10. hypothyroidism | j. of intestine |

**Task 9   Choose the right answer to fill in the blanks in the passage.**

For many years British people have been __1__ to eat at least "five-a-day"— that is five items of fruit or vegetables every day in order to improve their health and __2__ the likelihood of illness, in particular cancer.

The recommendation was first __3__ in 1990 by the World Health Organization which said that the "five-a-day" diet could prevent cancer and other chronic diseases. __4__ the advice has been a mainstay(支柱) of public health policies in many developed countries, such as the UK, __5__ the population eat a high proportion of junk food.

Many health campaigns have __6__ the advice, and indeed much food packaging in Britain states how the contents will constitute part of your five-a-day.

__7__, a study of 500,000 Europeans from 10 different countries refutes(驳斥) the commonly-believed suggestion that up to 50% of cancers could be prevented by __8__ the public's consumption of fruit and vegetables.

Instead the study, which is led by researchers from a well-respected New York medical school, estimated that only 2.5% of cancers could be averted by eating more fruit and vegetables.

It seems that the __9__ to avoid cancers is to have an overall healthy lifestyle which includes not smoking or drinking a lot of alcohol, taking exercise and avoiding obesity.

But medical charities have spoken out to __10__ people that diet is an important factor in staying healthy, and that even a 2.5% reduction in cancers is still a positive step.

1. A. compelled    B. recommended    C. proposed    D. required

Note

18

2. A. decline          B. undermine        C. destroy          D. reduce
3. A. put across       B. put down         C. put forward      D. put up
4. A. For the time     B. At present       C. Little by little D. Since then
5. A. where            B. when             C. that             D. which
6. A. mentioned        B. declared         C. promoted         D. reflected
7. A. Similarly        B. Though           C. Therefore        D. However
8. A. lessening        B. diminishing      C. increasing       D. rising
9. A. aim              B. key              C. objective        D. way
10. A. recall          B. propose          C. arouse           D. remind

## Part 4　Write and Learn

### Doctor's Certificate

**Direction**：Read the following writing samples carefully. Design and finish an imitated writing task with similar style.

诊　断　书

医生的诊断书包括患者姓名、年龄、入院时间、入院原因、治疗方式和时间、出院时间、建议休息时间等。

【Sample 1】

Doctor's Certificate

June 18<sup>th</sup>, 2012

This is to certify that the patient，Mr. Thomas，male，aged 41，was admitted into our hospital on June 9th，2012 for suffering from acute appendicitis. After immediate operation and ten days of treatment，he has got complete recovery and will be discharge on June 19th，2012. It is suggested that he should rest for one week at home before returning to his work.

(Signature) Jack Hopkins<br>Surgeon-in-chief

【Sample 2】

Doctor's Certificate

Feb 2<sup>nd</sup>, 2012

This is to certify that Ms. Zhou Xiumei has a high fever of 39 ℃ and a severe sore throat. We advise that she should take a three-day rest，and，if necessary，come back for a check by that time.

(Signature) Dong Yuxi<br>Physician-in-chief

【Assignment】

Write a doctor's certification according to the following information.

张明，男，21 岁，2012 年 3 月 5 日因腹泻住院，经一周治疗已痊愈，将于 3 月 12 日出院。医生建议他在家休息一周再上学。

*Note*

## Part 5  Prefixes, Suffixes & Roots

**Digestive System (消化系统)**

| 汉语(英语) | 常用词根 | 例　词 |
|---|---|---|
| 食管(esophagus) | esophag(o)- | esophagoscope 食管镜；gastroesophageal 胃食管的 |
| 胃(stomach) | gastr(o)-；stomach(o)- | gastritis 胃炎；gastroscopy 胃镜检查；gastropathy 胃病；stomachache 胃痛 |
| 肠(intestine) | enter(o)- | enteritis 肠炎；enterovirus 肠道病毒；enterobacteria 肠道菌；gastroenteritis 胃肠炎 |
| 十二指肠(duodenum) | duoden(o)- | duodenal 十二指肠的；gastroduodenal 胃十二指肠的 |
| 结肠(colon) | col(o)-；colon(o)- | colocentesis 结肠穿刺术；colitis 结肠炎；colonoscopy 结肠镜检查；paracolic 结肠周围的 |
| 消化(digestion) | peps(o)-；-gest(o)- | dyspepsia 消化不良；pepsin 胃蛋白酶；digestive 消化的；digestible 可消化的 |
| 直肠(rectum) | rect(o)-；procto- | rectocele 直肠膨出；rectouterine 直肠子宫肌；proctoptosis 直肠脱垂；proctoscopy 直肠镜检查 |
| 胆囊(gallbladder；cholecyst) | cholecyst(o)- | cholecystitis 胆囊炎；cholecystolithiasis/cholelithiasis 胆囊结石病(或胆石症) |
| 肝(liver) | hepat(o)- | hepatitis 肝炎；hepatorrhexis 肝破裂 |
| 胆管(bile duct) | cholangi(o)- | cholangitis 胆管炎；cholangiography 胆管造影术 |
| 阑尾(appendix) | appendic(o)- | appendicitis 阑尾炎；appendicectomy 阑尾切除术 |

**Task 10  Learn the prefixes, suffixes or roots in the table by heart and then choose the best answer to finish the exercises.**

1. The Chinese meaning for "pepsin" is _____.

A. 胃蛋白酶　　　　B. 胃泌素　　　　　C. 胃蛋白酶原　　　D. 胃酶抑素

2. Fill in the blank with the combining part for the medical term "结肠镜检查": _____ -scopy.

A. entero　　　　　B. recto　　　　　　C. colono　　　　　D. colo

3. The Chinese meaning for "cholecystitis" is _____.

A. 胆囊炎　　　　　B. 膀胱炎　　　　　C. 肝炎　　　　　　D. 胆管炎

4. The English term for "直肠脱垂" is _____.

A. rectouterine　　B. proctoptosis　　C. colitis　　　　　D. rectocele

5. The term "duodenum" is so called because it is about twelve _____.

A. fingerlengths　　　　　　　　　　　B. fingerbreadths

C. fingercircle　　　　　　　　　　　D. fingercircumferrence

6. The word which has nothing to do with liver is _____.

A. hepatitis　　　　B. hepatolithiasis　　C. hepatorrhexis　　D. pancreatitis

7. To make a word for "胆管造影术", its correct spelling is _____.

A. cholangiopancreatography      B. cholangiocarcinoma

C. cholangiography               D. cholecystectomy

8. The following words have the meaning of inflammation except _____.

A. pancreatitis      B. hepatitis      C. cholangitis      D. gastropathy

9. Which word has the meaning of "胆囊切除术"? _____

A. hepatolithiasis               B. cholecystectomy

C. cholecystolithiasis           D. cholecystoctomy

10. Which word has nothing to do with stomach? _____

A. gastritis      B. gastropathy      C. stomatitis      D. stomachache

# Unit 3　The Respiratory System

## Learning Objectives:

To remember some key English words related to the respiratory system.

To understand the conversation about admitting a patient and talk about the topic.

To read and understand the main ideas and the details of the passages about the respiratory system.

To learn to write discharge summary with the help of the given sample writing.

To learn by heart some word roots, prefixes and suffixes about the respiratory system.

## Part 1　Look and Learn

**Warming-up 1: Look at the following picture, talk about them and then finish Task 1.**

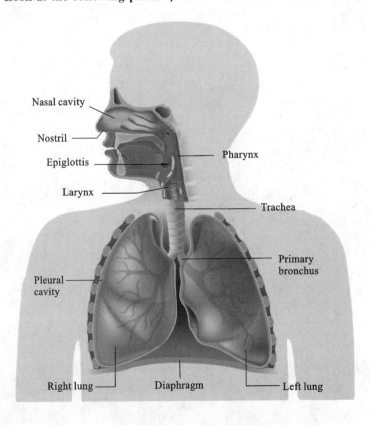

## New Words

nostril ['nɒstrəl] n. 鼻孔,鼻孔内壁

epiglottis [ˌepɪ'glɒtɪs] n. 会厌,喉头盖

pharynx ['færɪŋks] n. 咽

larynx ['lærɪŋks] n. 喉

trachea [trə'ki:ə] n. 气管,导管

pleural ['plʊrəl] adj. 肋膜的,胸膜的

bronchus ['brɒŋkəs] n.(尤指肺两侧的)支气管

diaphragm ['daɪəfræm] n. 横膈膜

**Task 1**　**Match the words in the left column with the explanations in the right column.**

| 1. diaphragm | A. a thin piece of tissue behind the tongue that prevents food or drink from entering the lungs |
|---|---|
| 2. trachea | B. either of the two openings at the end of the nose that you breathe through |
| 3. lung | C. the tube in the throat that carries air to the lungs |
| 4. epiglottis | D. either of the two organs in the chest that you use for breathing |
| 5. nostril | E. a muscular partition separating the abdominal and thoracic cavities; functions in respiration |

**Warming-up 2：Look at the following pictures about medical instruments, talk about them and then finish Task 2.**

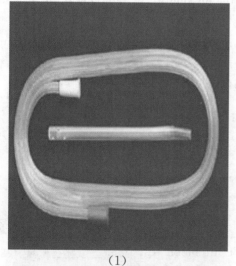

(1)

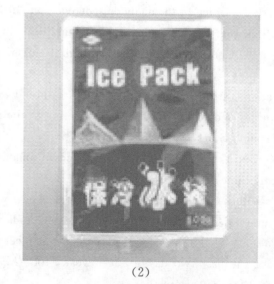

(2)

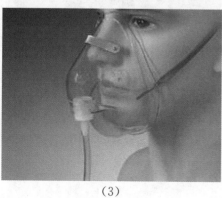

(3)

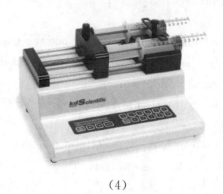

(4)

*Note*

## New Words

tube [tjuːb] n. 管，管状物

oxygen ['ɒksɪdʒən] n. 氧气

syringe ['sɪrɪndʒ] n. 注射器，注射筒

**Task 2　Match the picture number with the proper English and Chinese meaning.**

| Picture number | English | Chinese |
| --- | --- | --- |
| | syringe driver | 注射器泵 |
| | drain tube | 引流管 |
| | cold/hot pack | 冷/热敷袋 |
| | oxygen mask | 氧气面罩 |

# Part 2　Listen and Learn

## Situation Dialogue：Admitting a Patient

**Task 3　Listen to the audio episode one and fill in the missing words referring to the original text. Then check your writing against the original.**

Nurse：Good morning, Mrs. Wilson. I am the nurse of the 1._____. My name is Emily. I'll be 2._____ you to the ward today.

Patient：Good morning, Emily. What should I do now?

Nurse：Would you please come with me to the nurses' office so I can finish the paperwork first?

Patient：Sure. May I sit down?

Nurse：Yes, of course. Please sit down and make yourself comfortable, OK? Can you tell me your full name and your date of birth?

Patient：My full name is Rose Wilson. And I was born on 3._____, 1968.

Nurse：Can you tell me why you are here today?

Patient：Well, um. I've had a duodenal ulcer for about five years. My 4._____ have been black for the past two days. I feel weak, too. My occult blood test is 5._____, so my doctor suggested for me to come here.

**Task 4　Listen to the audio episode two and complete the answers according to the questions.**

1. What causes Mrs. Wilson's duodenal ulcer?

   It came from too much _____ in her job.

2. What's the result of Mrs. Wilson's BP?

   It's _____.

3. Why does Mrs. Wilson think her pulse is too fast?

   Because she always feels _____ these days.

扫码听
课文 A

# Part 3　Read and Learn

**Passage A**

## Common Cold

The common cold, also known as an upper respiratory tract infection, is a contagious illness that can be caused by a number of different types of viruses. Because of the great number of viruses that can cause a cold and because new cold viruses develop, the body never builds up resistance against all of them. For this reason, cold are a frequent and recurring problem.

Symptoms of a common cold include nasal stuffiness, drainage, sore throat, hoarseness, cough, and perhaps a fever and headache. Many people with colds feel tired and achy. These symptoms typically last from 3 to 10 days.

Colds often get better within a few days to weeks, whether or not you take medication. However, a cold virus can pave the way for other infections to invade the body, including sinus or ear infections, and bronchitis. If you have asthma, chronic bronchitis, or emphysema, your symptoms may be worsened for many weeks even after your cold has gone away.

The common cold is spread mostly by hand-to-hand contact. For example, a person with a cold blows or touches his or her nose and then touches someone else who then becomes infected with the virus. Additionally, the cold virus can live on objects such as pens, books, and coffee cups and can be acquired from such objects. While common sense would suggest that coughing and sneezing spread the common cold, these are actually very poor mechanisms for spreading a cold.

Generally antibiotics are not useful for treating a cold. Antibiotics only work against illnesses caused by bacteria and colds are often caused by viruses. Not only do antibiotics not help, but they can also cause allergic reactions that may be fatal. Further, using antibiotics when they are not necessary has led to the growth of several strains of common bacteria that have become resistant to antibiotics. For these and other reasons, it is important to limit the use of antibiotics to situations in which they are necessary. Sometimes, an infection with bacteria can follow the cold virus. Bacterial complications that arise from common cold are treated with antibiotics.

Several treatments that can ease the symptoms associated with a common cold also exist. Decongestants and nasal sprays can help reduce symptoms. People with heart disease, poorly controlled high blood pressure, or other illness should contact their physician prior to using these medications. Additionally, over-the-counter nasal sprays should not be used for more than three days because the nose can become dependent on them and a worse stuffy nose will result when they are discontinued.

## New Words

allergic [əˈlɜːdʒɪk] adj. 过敏的
antibiotic [ˌæntɪbaɪˈɒtɪk] n. 抗生素
　　　　　　　adj. 抗生素的
asthma [ˈæsmə] n. 哮喘
bacterial [bækˈtɪərɪəl] adj. 细菌的

*Note*

25

bronchitis [ brɒŋˈkaɪtɪs] n. 支气管炎

chronic [ˈkrɒnɪk] adj. 慢性的

complication [ˌkɒmplɪˈkeɪʃən] n. 并发症

contagious [ kənˈteɪdʒəs] adj. 传染性的，会感染的

decongestant [ˌdiːkənˈdʒestənt] n. 解充血药

drainage [ˈdreɪnɪdʒ ] n. 排水，引流

emphysema [ˌemfɪˈsiːmə ] n. 气肿，肺气肿

infection [ɪnˈfekʃən ] n. 传染，感染

mechanism [ˈmekənɪzəm] n. 机制

recur [ rɪˈkɜː(r) ] v. 复发

sinus [ˈsaɪnəs] n. 窦

spray [spreɪ] n. 喷雾，飞沫

tract [ trækt] n. 管道

virus [ˈvaɪrəs] n. 病毒

**Task 5　Fill in the blanks with the words given below and change the word forms if necessary.**

1. The _____(bacterial) are harmless to humans.

2. Foreign doctors and nurses are trying for instance, to stem the spread of _____ (infection) diseases.

3. Smoking also causes forty-two percent of cause of the chronic respiratory disease, including asthma, _____(bronchi) and emphysema.

4. These are classical examples of food _____(allergic).

5. Blindness is a common _____(complicate) of diabetes.

6. He experiences _____(chronic), almost pathological jealousy.

7. The case studies confirmed that many issues _____(recurrent).

8. The _____(contagious) of the virus will influence the speed of spread, both within countries and internationally.

9. The city planner decided to build an underground _____(drain) system.

10. That, in turn, boosted understanding of hepatitis B and hepatitis C and still other _____(virus).

**Task 6　Choose the correct answer according to the passage.**

1. Which of the followings is nothing to do with the common cold? _____

A. It is an upper respiratory tract infection

B. It is a contagious illness

C. It can be caused by coronavirus

D. It can be caused by a number of different types of viruses

2. Why is common cold a frequent and recurring problem? _____

A. Because the great number of viruses can cause a cold

B. Because new cold viruses develop

C. Because the body never builds up resistance against all of them

D. All of the above

3. What are the symptoms of the common cold? _____

Note

A. nasal stuffiness and drainage    B. sore throat

C. hoarseness    D. all of the above

4. Which is actually the common way for spreading a cold? _____

A. hand-to-hand contact    B. coughing

C. sneezing    D. all of the above

5. Which one can help reduce symptoms of a common cold? _____

A. sprays    B. decongestants

C. morphine    D. insulin

**Task 7  Arrange the following steps in proper sequence based on the medical procedure.**

_____ Very carefully build up pads of cotton wool around the object until they are at least the same height as the object. Do not pull the gauze down as you do this. If it is not possible to build up the dressing high enough, leave the embedded object protruding.

_____ Help the casualty lie down and raise and support the injured part. Drape a piece of gauze over the wound and object.

_____ Continue making these diagonal turns until the dressing is firm, and then secure the bandage.

_____ Control severe bleeding by pressing the area immediately above and below the object.

_____ Transfer the casualty to hospital.

_____ Pass the bandage under the limb and bring it up over the upper edge of the dressing.

## New Words

embed [ɪmˈbed] v. 把……嵌入

drape [dreɪp] v.(用布等)遮盖或装饰某人或某物

gauze [ɡɔːz] n. 纱布

protrude [prəˈtruːd] v.(使)突出,(使)伸出

immobilise [ɪˈməʊbɪlaɪz] v. 使不动,使不能移动

**Passage B**

### Bird Flu

Bird flu is also called avian flu, avian influenza and H5N1. "Bird flu" is a phrase similar to "Swine flu", "Dog flu", "Horse flu", or "Human flu" in that it refers to an illness caused by any of many different strains of influenza viruses that have adapted to a specific host.

Birds, just like people, get the flu. Bird flu viruses infect birds, including chickens, ducks, other poultry and wild birds. However, bird flu can pose health risks to people. The first case of the bird flu virus infecting a person directly, H5N1, was in Hong Kong,China in 1997. Since then, the bird flu virus has spread to birds in countries in Asia, Africa and Europe.

Human infection is still very rare, but the virus that causes the infection in birds might change, or mutate, to more easily infect humans. This could lead to a pandemic, or a worldwide outbreak of the illness.

During an outbreak of bird flu, people who have contact with infected birds can become sick. It may also be possible to catch bird flu by eating poultry that is not well cooked or through contact with a person who has it. Bird flu can make people very sick or even cause death. There is currently no

扫码听
课文 B

*Note*

27

vaccine.

Bird flu viruses occur naturally among birds. Wild birds worldwide carry the viruses in their intestines, but usually do not get sick from them. However, The viruses are very contagious among birds and can make some domesticated birds, including chickens, ducks and turkeys, very sick and kill them.

Infected birds shed influenza virus in their saliva, nasal secretions, and feces. Susceptible birds become infected when they have contact with contaminated secretions or excretions or with surfaces that are contaminated with secretions or excretions from infected birds. Domesticated birds may become infected with the virus through direct contact with infected waterfowl or other infected poultry, or through contact with surfaces (such as dirt or cages) or materials (such as water or feed) that have been contaminated with the virus.

Symptoms of bird flu in humans have ranged from typical human influenza-like symptoms (fever, cough, sore throat, muscle aches, etc.) to eye infections, pneumonia, severe respiratory diseases (such as acute respiratory distress), and other severe and life-threatening complications. The symptoms of bird flu may depend on which virus caused the infection.

Studies done in laboratories suggest that some of the prescription medicines should work in treating bird flu infection in humans. However, influenza viruses can become resistant to these medications, so these medications may not always work. Additional studies are needed to demonstrate the effectiveness of these medications.

## New Words

avian ['eɪvɪən] adj. 鸟类的
                  n. 鸟

contaminate [kən'tæmɪneɪt] v. 污染

domesticate [dəʊ'mestɪkeɪt] v. 驯养，使安于土地，教化

feces ['fiːsiːz] n. 粪，屎，渣滓

host [həʊst] n. 宿主

influenza [ˌɪnflʊ'enzə] n. 流行性感冒

mutate [mjuː'teɪt] v. 变异

poultry ['pəʊltrɪ] n. 家禽

vaccine ['væksiːn] adj. 疫苗的，牛痘的
                  n. 疫苗

intestine [ɪn'testɪn] n. 肠

prescription [prɪ'skrɪpʃən] n. 处方，药方

resistant [rɪ'zɪstənt] adj. 有耐药性的

saliva [sə'laɪvə] n. 口水，唾液

secretion [sɪ'kriːʃən] n. 分泌，分泌物（液）

susceptible [sə'septəbl] adj. 易受影响的
                  n. （因缺乏免疫力）易患病的人

## Exercises

**Task 8  Match the words or phrases with similar meaning in the two columns.**

| A | B |
|---|---|
| 1. isolate | a. death rate |
| 2. hepatitis | b. muscle pain |
| 3. mutate | c. pollute |
| 4. sore | d. doctor's order for the use of a medicine |
| 5. myalgia | e. liver trouble |
| 6. mortality | f. change |
| 7. host | g. separate |
| 8. prescription | h. aching |
| 9. poultry | i. animals or plants on which a parasite lives |
| 10. contaminate | j. domesticated bird |

**Task 9  Choose the right answer to fill in the blanks in the passage.**

Patricia Turse has seen what music can do. As a __1__ music therapist, Patricia spends her days working with children to make them __2__ afraid and more comfortable while they're in the hospital. Music was always part of her life and she wanted to do something __3__ with her talent. "I wanted to help people and music was always beneficial for me. I was convinced that it could be __4__ in many ways," says Patricia. Patricia currently works with children, but she has also treated __5__ and chemically addicted adults. She sees 10 to 15 children a day on a one-to-one basis since each child has a different set of needs to be addressed. "I help them manage pain, separation or anxiety. Sometimes I only get one day to get to know and __6__ a child before he or she goes home," states Patricia. "I feel like I have something to give by using music to calm and heal others." Patricia may play the harp for them or teach breathing techniques to help them deal with __7__ they're going through. "Sometimes we sing or they write a song with me," says Patricia. She recalls treating a 5-year old girl who had autism. "She loved drumming so we sang and __8__ all day. She didn't want to give up the drum at the end of the session. I really enjoyed her. __9__ can help to improve a child's __10__ and socialization skills," notes Patricia. Patty certainly helps to add beautiful notes to these children's lives.

1. A. certify       B. certificate       C. certified        D. certificated
2. A. more         B. less              C. much            D. little
3. A. special      B. more              C. important        D. vital
4. A. useless      B. helpless          C. useful           D. helpful
5. A. psychologically ill               B. chemically ill
   C. physically ill                    D. mentally ill
6. A. to access    B. access            C. close            D. to close
7. A. whatever     B. which             C. that             D. what
8. A. drumming     B. drum              C. drummed          D. drums
9. A. Music therapy  B. Chemotherapy    C. Physiotherapy    D. Therapy
10. A. abilities    B. talent           C. communication    D. music skills

*Note*

# Part 4　Write and Learn

## Discharge Summary

**Direction**：**Read the following writing sample carefully. Design and finish an imitated writing task with similar style.**

与其他应用文相比,写病情报告、病例等短文时一般会提供较为详细的信息,学生只要连词成句即可。写作时常用一般现在时、现在完成时和一般过去时;同时也常使用被动语态。

【Sample】

Patient's name：Peter Morgan

Sex：Male

Occupation：Driver

DOB：Oct. 5th, 1980

Chief complaint：Fever for 3 days, got worse today; seizure at home this morning

History：Oral ulcer noted for 3 days

　　　　Hands, legs and buttock rash noted for 2 days

　　　　Activity and appetite normal in the first few days

　　　　Vomiting since this morning

　　　　Mild headache

The patient's name is Peter Morgan, male, 30 years old, and is currently a driver for a living. He got a fever 3 days ago and became worse today. Moreover, he has attacked by a seizure at home this morning. He has suffered oral ulcer for 3 days, and rash can be seen on his hands, legs, and buttock. His activity and appetite are both normal in the first few days, but he vomited a number of times since this morning. He also complained about a mild headache.

【Assignment】

Read the patient discharge summary. Use the information in the summary to write a case report in about 100 words.

| Discharge Summary | |
|---|---|
| **Patient**：Mrs. Martha | **DOB**：17/9/21 |
| **Date of discharge**：May 10th, 2009 | **Date of admission**：April 23rd, 2009 |

**Problems**：
Has been suffering from hypertension & degenerative bone disease
Needs to urinate frequently
Diagnosed：left pneumonia & urinary tract infection

**Next of kin**：
No immediate family

**Needs**：
Bath seat and safety rails in bathroom
Nurse to visit 2 weeks to monitor medications
Physiotherapy 3 weeks

*Note*

续表

| Discharge Summary | | |
|---|---|---|
| **Strengths and resources:** | | |
| Independent-minded woman, fully alert and articulate, can cook | | |

# Part 5　Prefixes, Suffixes & Roots

## Respiratory System (呼吸系统)

| 汉语(英语) | 常用词根 | 例　词 |
|---|---|---|
| 呼吸(breath) | -pnea; pneum(o)-; -spir(o) | expiration 呼气;inspiration 吸气; tachypnea 呼吸过速;bradypnea 呼吸过缓; dyspnea 呼吸困难;pneumothorax 气胸 |
| 鼻(nose) | rhin(o)-; naso- | rhinitis 鼻炎;rhinorrhoea 鼻漏;nasobronchial 鼻支气管; nasoscope 鼻镜;endonasopharyngeal 鼻咽内的 |
| 喉(larynx) | laryng(o)- | laryngitis 喉炎;laryngectomy 喉切除术 |
| 咽(pharynx) | pharyng(o)- | pharyngeal 咽部;pharyngitis 咽炎;pharyngoplasty 咽成形术; rhinopharynx 鼻咽 |
| 气管(windpipe) | trach(o)-; trache(o)- | tracheotomy 气管切开术;trachitis 气管炎;tracheobronchitis 气管支气管炎 |
| 支气管(bronchi) | bronch(o)- | bronchiectasis 支气管扩张;bronchitis 支气管炎;bronchoscope 支气管镜;bronchogenic 支气管原的 |
| 肺(lung) | pneumon(o)-; pulmo(n)- | pneumonia 肺炎;bronchopneumonia 支气管肺炎;pulmonary 肺的;bronchopulmonary 支气管肺的 |
| 胸膜(pleura) | pleur(o)- | pleuritis 胸膜炎;pleural 胸膜的 |

**Task 10　Learn the prefixes, suffixes or roots in the table by heart and then choose the best answer to finish the exercises.**

1. The word "windpipe" is related to _____.

A. trachy-　　　　B. trachelo-　　　　C. teacho-　　　　D. tracheo-

2. In medical term, the combining form strictly related to "larynx" is _____.

A. laryngo-　　　　B. larygo-　　　　C. pharyngo-　　　　D. pharygo-

3. Which word in the following has nothing to do with "breath"?_____

A. inspiration　　　B. spirochaeta　　　C. expiration　　　D. respiration

4. The correct spelling form for "支气管炎" is _____.

A. bronchoitis　　　B. brancheitis　　　C. bronchitis　　　D. bronchoeitis

5. Which word in the following represents the abnormal respiration?_____

A. pneumoperitonue　B. orthopnea　　　C. expiration　　　D. pneumaturia

6. The combining form "spiro-" is related to _____.

A. breath　　　　B. air　　　　C. lung　　　　D. chest

7. The combining form only denoting relationship to "lung" is _____.

*Note*

A. pleur(o)-        B. pneumati-        C. pneumono-        D. alve(o)-

8. The English term for "气管切开术" is _____.

A. tracheotomy        B. tracheoectomy        C. bronchiectomy        D. bronchoectomy

9. The word "breath" is not related to _____.

A. pneum(o)-        B. -spir(o)        C. pneumon(o)-        D. -pnea

10. The expression for lung function which is used most often is _____.

A. pneumonofunction                B. pneumofunction

C. pulmonary function              D. pulmofunction

# Unit 4　The Nervous System

## Learning Objectives:

To remember some key English words related to the nervous system.

To understand the conversation in the nurses' office and talk about the topic.

To read and understand the main ideas and the details of the passages about the nervous system.

To learn to write a history of illness with the help of the given sample writing.

To learn by heart some word roots, prefixes and suffixes about the nervous system.

## Part 1　Look and Learn

**Warming-up 1: Look at the following pictures, talk about them and then finish Task 1.**

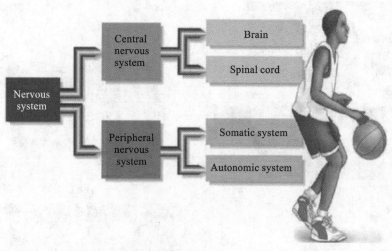

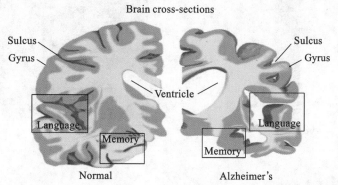

Brain cross-sections

*Note*

## New Words & Phrases

peripheral [pəˈrɪfərəl] adj. 外围的,(神经)末梢区域的

　　　　　　　　n. 外部设备

spinal cord [ˈspaɪnəl kɔːd] 脊髓

somatic [səʊˈmætɪk] adj. 躯体的,身体的

autonomic [ˌɔːtəˈnɒmɪk] adj. 自主的,不受意志支配的

ventricle [ˈventrɪkl] n. 脑室,心室

sulcus [ˈsʌlkəs] n. 脑沟

gyrus [ˈdʒaɪrəs] n. 脑回

**Task 1　Match the words in the left column with the explanations in the right column.**

| 1. brain | A. one of the small bones that form the spine |
|---|---|
| 2. nerve | B. the organ inside the head that controls thought，memory，feeling and activity |
| 3. spinal cord | C. a group of long thin fibers that carry information or instructions between the brain and other parts of the body |
| 4. skull | D. the set of nerves inside the spine that connect the brain to other nerves in the body |
| 5. vertebra | E. the bones of the head，which surround the brain and give the head shape |

**Warming-up 2: Look at the following pictures about medical instruments, talk about them and then finish Task 2.**

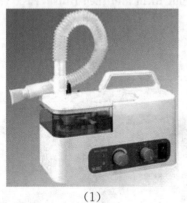

(1)

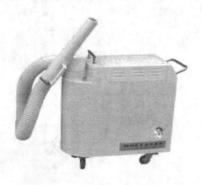

(2)

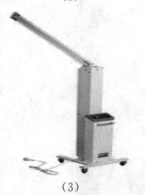

(3)

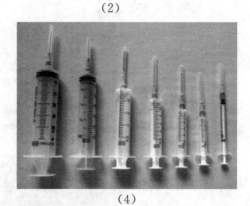

(4)

*Note*

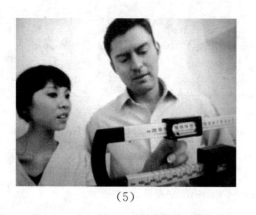
(5)

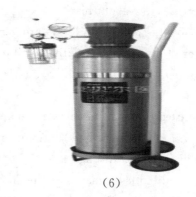
(6)

## New Words

nebulizer ['nebjʊlaɪzə(r)] n. 喷雾器

sterilization [ˌsterəlaɪ'zeɪʃən] n. 杀菌，绝育

hypodermic [ˌhaɪpə'dɜːmɪk] adj. 皮下注射用的

ultraviolet [ˌʌltrə'vaɪələt] adj. 紫外的，紫外线的

n. 紫外线

**Task 2    Match the picture number with the proper English and Chinese meaning.**

| Picture number | English | Chinese |
|---|---|---|
| | air sterilization machine | 空气消毒机 |
| | ultraviolet sterilizer | 紫外线消毒器 |
| | hypodermic syringe | 皮下注射器 |
| | scale | 秤 |
| | oxygen tank | 氧气罐 |
| | nebulizer | 喷雾器 |

# Part 2    Listen and Learn

## Situation Dialogue：In the Nurses' Office

**Task 3    Listen to the audio episode one and fill in the missing words referring to the original text. Then check your writing against the original.**

Doctor：Hello. Mary, are you looking after Mr. John today?

Nurse：Yes. Any question?

Doctor：Oh, can we take a few minutes to talk about his situation?

Nurse：Sure. Have a seat, please.

Doctor：Thank you. He was back from the OR an hour ago and there are a lot of orders for him. Let's make sure they are clear.

Nurse：OK. Let me see. 1. _____ every 30 minutes, temperature every 4 hours. And monitor the GCS every 4 hours.

Doctor：And also monitor his I & O, OK?

扫码听
对话 1

*Note*

Nurse: Sure. How about his 2. _____?

Doctor: Now his potassium levels are very low according to his blood result. Would you please give him a liter of normal saline with 20 millimoles of KCl?

Nurse: Sure. Please fill out the patient's 3. _____ first.

**Task 4  Listen to the audio episode two and complete the answers according to the questions.**

1. How will the nurse run the antibiotics for Mr. John?

   She will run them through a _____.

2. Besides antibiotics, what does the doctor want to give to Mr. John?

   He wants to give him some _____ with the fluids.

3. Why can these nutrients not be run through the cannula?

   Because these nutrients are _____, and it's easy to cause _____.

扫码听
对话 2

# Part 3   Read and Learn

**Passage A**

**Introduction to the Brain and the Nervous System**

**The brain & the nervous system in everyday life**

If the brain is like a central computer that controls all the functions of the body, then the nervous system is like a network that sends messages back and forth from the brain to different parts of the body. It does this via the spinal cord, which runs from the brain down through the back and contains threadlike nerves that branch out to every organ and tissue of the body.

When a message comes into the brain from anywhere in the body, the brain tells the body how to react. For example, if you accidentally touch a hot stove, the nerves in your skin shoot a message of pain to your brain. Your brain then sends a message back telling the muscles in your hands to pull away. Luckily, this neurological relay race takes a lot less time than it just took to read about it!

**How the brain works**

Considering everything it does, the human brain is incredibly compact, weighing just 3 pounds. Its many folds and grooves, provide it with the additional surface area necessary for storing all of the body's important information.

The spinal cord is a long bundle of nerve tissue about 18 inches long and a 3/4 inch thick. It extends from the lower part of the brain down through spine. Along the way, various nerves branch out to the entire body. These make up the peripheral nervous system.

Both the brain and the spinal cord are protected by bones. The brain by the bones of the skull, and the spinal cord by the set of ring-shaped bones called vertebrae that make up the spine. They're both cushioned by layers of membranes called meninges as well as a special fluid called cerebrospinal fluid. This fluid helps protect the nerve tissue, keep it healthy, and remove waste products.

## New Words

nervous [ˈnɜːvəs] adj. 紧张的,神经的

accidentally [ˌæksɪˈdentəlɪ] adv. 意外地

neurological [ˌnjʊərəˈlɒdʒɪkəl] adj. 神经学的,神经科的

*Note*

incredibly [ɪnˈkredəblɪ] adv. 难以置信地

compact [kəmˈpækt，ˈkɒmpækt] adj. 紧凑的，紧密的

                      n. 带镜小粉盒，协定

groove [gruːv] n. 沟，槽，音乐节奏

              v. 在……开沟，跟着流行乐跳舞，过得快活

peripheral [pəˈrɪfərəl] adj. 次要的，周边的，与计算机相连的

                  n. 外围设备

cushion [ˈkʊʃən] n. 软垫，坐垫，靠垫

            v. 缓和冲击（用垫子）使柔和

layer [ˈleɪə(r)] n. 层

         v. 分层堆放

membrane [ˈmembreɪn] n. （身体内）膜，（植物）细胞膜，（可起防水作用等的）膜状物

meninges [mɪˈnɪndʒiːz] n. 脑膜

cerebrospinal [ˌserɪbrəʊˈspaɪnəl] adj. 脑脊髓的

fluid [ˈfluːɪd] n. 液体，流体

        adj. 流畅优美的，易变的，流动的，流体的

**Task 5  Fill in the blanks with the words given below and change the word forms if necessary.**

1. When you practicing shooting, you are supposed to aim at and focus on the _____ (central) of the target.

2. The expectant mother was _____ (nerve), stressful and scary before she delivered her baby.

3. The dietitian is explaining to the patients that they could prevent the disease by eating foods _____ (contain) rich vitamins.

4. The survivors in the traffic _____ (accidentally) were severely injured and sent to the first aid center.

5. The diagnosis from the _____ (neurological) showed that he suffered from a chronic disease related to the nervous system.

6. The child's performance is _____ (incredible) outstanding in the swimming contest.

7. The physically inactive patient had an _____ (health) diet and he did no exercises.

8. An ovary is a woman's organ in the _____ (product) system while a penis is a man's organ.

9. Elimination is an essential part of human being's physiological process, which mainly deals with the _____ (remove) of wastes produced by the body.

10. The science of medicine is traditionally classified in basic medicine, _____ (prevention) medicine, clinical medicine and rehabilitation medicine.

**Task 6  Choose the correct answer according to the passage.**

1. What is the brain compared to at the beginning of the text? _____

  A. an internet      B. a fishing net      C. a software      D. a central computer

2. Why can the spinal cord help us send messages back and forth from the brain to the different parts of the body? _____

  A. Because it controls all the functions of the body

  B. Because it runs from the head to the toe

*Note*

C. Because it has small nerves that extend to every organ and tissue of the body

D. Because it works as a central computer

3. What is protected by bone? _____

A. the brain      B. the spinal cord      C. neither A nor B      D. both A and B

4. Which of the following statements is true according to the passage? _____

A. The brain tells the body how to respond whenever a message comes into the brain

B. Once you unintentionally touch a hot stove, the nerves in your brain shoot a message of pain to your skin

C. The peripheral nervous system will send a message back telling the muscles in your hands to stay away from the fire if your hand is burnt

D. The neurological message relay usually takes a lot of time

5. Which is NOT true about cerebrospinal fluid according to the last paragraph in this passage? _____

A. It is something that helps protect the brain instead of the spinal cord

B. It is not a layer of membranes

C. This special fluid can promote the health of the nerve tissue

D. It helps get rid of unwanted materials which are not useful in the body

**Task 7** **Arrange the following steps about eye injury in proper sequence based on the medical procedure.**

_____ Support casualty's head: Support casualty's head to keep it as still as possible, and ask casualty to try not to move eyes.

_____ Wait for an ambulance.

_____ Place dressing over eye: Place a sterile pad or dressing over injured eye, ask casualty to hold this in place, and bandage dressing in place to cover injured eye. If embedded object in eye, lie casualty on back, place pad around object and bandage in place.

_____ Flush eye with cool and flowing water: If chemical or heat burn, or smoke in eyes, flush with water.

## New Words

sterile ['steraɪl] adj. 无菌的

pad [pæd] n. 垫,衬垫

flush [flʌʃ] v. (以水)冲刷,冲洗

**Passage B**

### Brain PET Scan

A brain positron emission tomography (PET) scan is an imaging test of the brain. It uses a radioactive substance called tracer to look for disease or injury in the brain. A PET scan shows how the brain and its tissues work. Other imaging tests, such as magnetic resonance imaging (MRI) and computed tomography (CT) scans only reveal the structure of the brain.

A PET scan requires a small amount of radioactive material (tracer). This tracer is given through a vein, usually near the elbow. The tracer travels through the blood and stops in the organs and tissues. The tracer helps the doctor, usually a radiologist, to see certain areas or diseases more clearly.

扫码听
课文 B

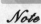

Note

The patients lie on a narrow table, which slides into a large tunnel-shaped scanner. The PET scanner detects the tracer in the organs and tissues. A computer changes the results into 3D pictures. The images are displayed on a monitor for the doctor or nurse to read.

This test has the following uses.

• Diagnose cancer and malignant tumors.

• Prepare for epilepsy surgery.

• Help diagnose dementia or Alzheimer's disease.

• Tell the differences between Parkinson disease and other movement disorders.

Several PET scans may be taken to determine how well you are responding to the treatment for cancer or another illness. The test takes between 30 minutes and 2 hours.

## New Words

positron ['pɒzɪtrɒn] n. 正电子,阳电子

emission [ɪ'mɪʃən] n. 射出,排放物

tomography [təʊ'mɒgrəfɪ] n. 体层摄影(利用 X 线和超声波清晰显示体内结构)

radioactive [ˌreɪdɪəʊ'æktɪv] adj. 放射性的,有辐射的

substance ['sʌbstəns] n. 物质,事实基础,要点,实质内容

tracer ['treɪsə(r)] n. 曳光弹,示踪剂,同位素指示剂

resonance ['rezənəns] n. 洪亮,响亮,共鸣,共振,谐振

radiologist [ˌreɪdɪ'ɒlədʒɪst] n. 放射科医生

tunnel ['tʌnəl] n. 隧道,挖隧道

malignant [mə'lɪgnənt] adj. 恶性的,恶意的

epilepsy ['epɪlepsɪ] n. 癫痫

dementia [dɪ'menʃə] n. 痴呆,精神错乱

## Exercises

**Task 8   Match the words or phrases with similar meaning in the two columns.**

|   A   |   B   |
|-------|-------|
| 1. emission | a. not wide |
| 2. malignant | b. disorder |
| 3. substance | c. show |
| 4. surgery | d. find |
| 5. respond | e. react |
| 6. determine | f. make clear |
| 7. detect | g. material |
| 8. display | h. operation |
| 9. disease | i. gas or heat sent out |
| 10. narrow | j. not benign |

**Task 9   Choose the right answer to fill in the blanks in the passage.**

Ten-year-old Benjamin Oback has the typical face of swine flu in its more serious stages. He lies in the ___1___ care unit at Davis Children's Hospital. His parents pray. For nearly two weeks, their son has been ___2___ for his life.

It started out like a normal ___3___. On Sunday, Oct. 4th, after riding his bike, Benjamin felt out

*Note*

39

of breath.

"On Sunday, he __4__ his chest hurt. He was seen to have a minor case of the flu." his mother Julie Oback said. "His __5__ listened to his lungs and said his lungs were __6__. I asked him about giving my son Tamiflu, but he said, 'No, he's not that sick. He should be better by the end of the week.' Nine hours later, he took a turn for the worse."

Benjamin had passed out and was rushed to the hospital.

"So that night, Tuesday night and early Wednesday morning was the worst." said Julie Oback. "This wasn't the normal __7__. Most people who get H1N1 are fine, but you don't know who's going to take a turn for the worse. That's what's so scary about it."

"In Benjamin's case, the main __8__ was that fluid built up on the outside of his lung rather than the inside of his lung, and I think that's probably why his pediatrician didn't catch it with a stethoscope." Benjamin's father said.

Already, H1N1 is proving far more deadly for children than the __9__ flu.

"When Benjamin first presented to the hospital, he was gravely ill." said Dr. Joanne Natale, who treated Benjamin. "He wasn't conscious. Now, he's __10__ significantly."

1. A. intensive      B. extensive      C. intense      D. extension
2. A. saving         B. facing         C. fighting     D. dying
3. A. influence      B. flue           C. flu          D. flux
4. A. explained      B. complained     C. explanation  D. complaint
5. A. surgeon        B. radiologist    C. pediatrician D. dermatologist
6. A. clear          B. pretty         C. injured      D. wounded
7. A. curse          B. course         C. record       D. recording
8. A. symptom        B. illness        C. injury       D. treatment
9. A. reason         B. reasonable     C. season       D. seasonal
10. A. recovered     B. uncovered      C. discovered   D. covered

## New Words & Phrases

complaint [kəmˈpleɪnt] n. 主诉
pediatrician [ˌpiːdɪəˈtrɪʃən] n. 小儿科医生
stethoscope [ˈsteθəskəʊp] n. 听诊器
prognosis [prɒɡˈnəʊsɪs] n. （对病情的）预断，预后
Tamiflu n. 特敏福（药品名称）
swine flu 猪流感
minor case 病情较轻的病例
intensive care unit 重症监护病房

## Part 4  Write and Learn

### History of Illness

**Direction: Read the following writing sample carefully. Design and finish an imitated writing task with similar style.**

病史是患者病程记录的第一部分。它由六个部分组成：主诉、现病史、过去史、家族史、社会史和系

统复习(系统回顾)。写病史时应基本掌握本专业内可能有的常用词汇和表达;在转述患者的话语时,一定要注意时态的正确运用。

【Sample】

## XXX Hospital

Patient's name:

Chart number:

Date of birth:

Sex:

Race:

Date of examination: mm/dd/yy

Date of admission: mm/dd/yy

Chief complaint:

Present illness:

Past history:

Family history:

Review of systems:

Impressions:

【Assignment】

Write a history of illness according to the following information.

## 滨江市第一医院住院部

患者姓名:约翰

病历号:15672

出生日期:1993 年 6 月 4 日

出生地点:美国纽约

性别:男

入院日期:2006 年 6 月 7 日

主诉:咳嗽,哮喘伴呼吸困难。

现病史:此次入院为该患者(13 岁)首次住院。患者从 3 岁开始有哮喘,但未住院治疗。入境后状态良好,入院前游长城发生气短,使用止咳药无效。哮喘逐渐加重,该患者被送往滨江市第一医院急症室,接受肾上腺素和氧气治疗,然后送回希尔顿饭店。3 h 后,该患者又被送往急症室并住院。

过去史:该患者 8 个半月时出生。免疫接种:完全。过敏史:灰尘,洋葱。

家族史:母亲 37 岁,父亲 40 岁,均健在。兄弟姐妹均身体健康。家族中无哮喘史及糖尿病史。

系统复习:除随时有结膜炎及哮喘外,其他为阴性。

诊断:支气管哮喘。

# Part 5 Prefixes, Suffixes & Roots

### Nervous System（神经系统）

| 汉语(英语) | 常用词根 | 例　词 |
|---|---|---|
| 脑(brain) | encephal(o)- | encephalitis 脑炎;encephalopathy 脑病;encephalomyelitis 脑脊髓炎 |

*Note*

续表

| 汉语（英语） | 常 用 词 根 | 例 词 |
|---|---|---|
| 大脑（cerebrum） | cerebr(o)- | cerebral 大脑的；cerebrovascular 脑血管的 |
| 小脑（cerebellum） | cerebell(o)- | archicerebellum 原小脑；cerebrocerebellum 皮层小脑 |
| 丘脑（thalamus） | thalam(o)- | metathalamus 后丘脑；epithalamus 上丘脑 |
| 髓质（marrow） | medull(o)- | medullary 髓质的；adrenomedullin 肾上腺髓质素 |
| 脑膜,脊膜（membrane） | mening(o)- | meningitis 脑膜炎；leptomeningitis 软脑膜炎；pachymeningitis 硬脑膜炎 |
| 脊柱（spine） | spin(o)- | spinocerebellum 脊柱小脑；cerebrospinal 脑脊的 |
| 精神,意志（mind） | psych(o)- | psychopathology 精神病理学；psychostimulant 精神兴奋剂 |
| 神经（nerve） | neur(o)- | neurology 神经病学；neurotmesis 神经断伤 |
| 蛛网膜（arachnoid） | arachn (o)- | arachnoidal 蛛网膜的；arachnoiditis 蛛网膜炎；subarachnoid 蛛网膜下 |
| 狂,癖（madness） | -mania(c) | erotomania 色情狂；tocomania 产后躁狂；dipsomania 酒狂 |

**Task 10　Learn the prefixes, suffixes or roots in the table by heart and then choose the best answer to finish the exercises.**

1. Which is the correct meaning of the term "脑血管的"：_____ vascular?

A. encephalo-　　　B. brain　　　C. cerebro-　　　D. cerebello-

2. The term "leptomeningitis" can be translated into Chinese term _____.

A. 脑膜炎　　　B. 软脑膜炎　　　C. 硬脑膜炎　　　D. 脑膜膨出

3. The correct Chinese meaning of the word "arachnoid" is _____.

A. 蛛网膜下　　　B. 蛛网膜炎　　　C. 蛛网膜下腔　　　D. 蛛网膜

4. The word "subthalamus" means the portion situated _____ the thalamus.

A. above　　　B. over　　　C. under　　　D. near

5. The branch of medical science that is concerned with nerves is termed as _____.

A. neurology　　　B. neuroscience　　　C. neurobranch　　　D. nervescience

6. Any degenerative disease of the brain is termed as _____.

A. encephalitis　　　B. encephaloma　　　C. leukoencephalitis　　　D. encephalopathy

7. What does the inflammation in both the brain and the spinal cord mean in medicine? _____

A. encephalomyelitis　B. leukoencephalitis　C. encephalalitis　　　D. cerebrospinauid

8. The combining part "encephalo-" denotes the relationship to the _____.

A. brain stem　　　B. brain　　　C. large brain　　　D. small brain

9. The combining part which denotes relationship to the membranes covering the brain is _____.

A. encephalo-　　　B. cerebro-　　　C. meningo-　　　D. cerebello-

10. Which combining part in the choice denotes the relationship to the madness? _____

A. -kinesia　　　B. -gnosis　　　C. -phobia　　　D. -mania

# Unit 5　The Endocrine and Lymphatic Systems

## Learning Objectives:

To remember some key English words related to the endocrine and lymphatic systems.

To understand the conversation about administering medications and talk about the topic.

To read and understand the main ideas and the details of the passages about the endocrine and lymphatic systems.

To learn to write a prescription with the help of the given sample writing.

To learn by heart some word roots, prefixes and suffixes about the endocrine and lymphatic systems.

## Part 1　Look and Learn

**Warming-up 1: Look at the following picture, talk about them and then finish Task 1.**

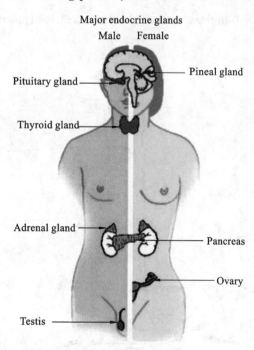

Major endocrine glands
Male　Female

Pituitary gland — Pineal gland
Thyroid gland
Adrenal gland — Pancreas
— Ovary
Testis

*Note*

## New Words

gland [glænd] n. 腺

pineal ['pɪnɪəl] adj. 松果体的

pituitary [pɪ'tjuːɪtərɪ] n. （脑）垂体

adj. 脑垂体的

thyroid ['θaɪrɔɪd] n. 甲状腺

adj. 甲状腺的

adrenal [ə'driːnəl] adj. 肾上腺的

n. 肾上腺

pancreas ['pæŋkrɪəs] n. 胰腺

ovary ['əʊvərɪ] n. 卵巢

testis ['testɪs] n. 睾丸（复数形式：testes）

**Task 1  Match the words in the left column with the explanations in the right column.**

| | |
|---|---|
| 1. pineal gland | A. a gland that is attached to the base of the brain, and produces hormones that affect growth, sexual development, and other functions of the body |
| 2. pituitary gland | B. an organ in the body that is situated behind the stomach, and produces insulin and substances that help the body digest food |
| 3. thyroid gland | C. a pea-sized organ in the brain, that secretes melatonin into the bloodstream |
| 4. adrenal gland | D. a gland in the neck that produces chemicals which control the way the body grows and functions |
| 5. pancreas | E. either of a pair of complex endocrine glands situated near the kidney |

**Warming-up 2：Look at the following picture about medical instruments, talk about them and then finish Task 2.**

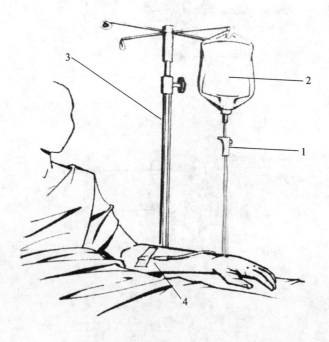

## New Words

clamp [klæmp] n. 钳，夹子

IV (abbr. intravenous) [ˌɪntrəˈviːnəs] adj. 静脉注射的

solution [səˈluːʃən] n. 溶液

catheter [ˈkæθɪtə(r)] n. 导管

**Task 2　Label the picture using the words in the box.**

| | |
| --- | --- |
| roller clamp(轮钳) | IV stand(静脉输液架) |
| IV solution bag(静脉输液药袋) | catheter(输液管，导管) |

1. _____

2. _____

3. _____

4. _____

# Part 2　Listen and Learn

## Situation Dialogue：Administering Medications

**Task 3　Listen to the audio episode one and fill in the missing words referring to the original text. Then check your writing against the original.**

Nurse：Hi，Janice. Good to see you again.

Patient：Thank you and me too. You look so nice today.

Nurse：How are you doing today?

Patient：Not good，I have a 1. _____ and feel 2. _____ today. My blood pressure was eighty over one ten (180/110) this morning. That's really high，isn't it?

Nurse：Oh，I see. That's the reason why Dr. Peter 3. _____ two new medications for you. One is metoprolol，to 4. _____ your BP. And another is Lasix，a diuretic.

Patient：Oh，I can't remember the names. Would you please repeat them?

Nurse：Sure，and I'll tell more about them. Metoprolol is in the green box，and I already wrote down the 5. _____ for you. You take this 2 pills once，twice a day，that's 8：00 am before your breakfast and 8：00 pm before your bedtime. Got it?

Patient：Mm，but I have a very poor memory. Instructions on the box are good for me.

扫码听
对话1

**Task 4　Listen to the audio episode two and complete the answers according to the questions.**

1. Why should the patient put this medication in a cool place?

   Because it would be _____ at 45 ℃.

2. What's the function of Lasix?

   It prevents our body from _____ too much _____ .

3. What's the nurse's suggestion for diet?

   The patient would better eat diet with more _____ .

扫码听
对话2

*Note*

# Part 3　Read and Learn

Passage A

## The Endocrine and Lymphatic Systems

**What is the endocrine system?**

Although we rarely think about the endocrine system, it influences almost every cell, organ, and function of our bodies. The endocrine system plays a role in regulating mood, growth and development, tissue function, metabolism, and sexual function and reproductive processes.

In general, the endocrine system is in charge of body processes that happen slowly, such as cell growth. Faster processes like breathing and body movement are controlled by the nervous system. But even though the nervous system and endocrine system are separate systems, they often work together to help the body functions properly.

The foundations of the endocrine system are the hormones and glands. As the body's chemical messengers, hormones transfer information and instructions from one set of cells to another. Many different hormones move through the bloodstream, but each type of hormone is designed to affect only certain cells. A gland is a group of cells that produces and secretes, or gives off chemicals. A gland selects and removes materials from the blood, processes them, and secretes the finished chemical products for use somewhere in the body.

**What is the lymphatic system?**

The lymphatic system is an extensive drainage network that helps keep bodily fluid levels in balance and defends the body against infections. The lymphatic system is made up of a network of lymphatic vessels. These vessels carry lymph — a clear and watery fluid containing proteins, salts, glucose, urea, and other substances — throughout the body. The spleen is located in the upper left part of the abdomen under the ribcage. It works as a part of the lymphatic system to protect the body, clearing worn-out red blood cells and other foreign bodies from the bloodstream to help fight off infection.

## New Words

endocrine ['endəʊkrɪn] adj. 内分泌的

lymphatic [lɪm'fætɪk] adj. 淋巴的

metabolism [mɪ'tæbəlɪzəm] n. 新陈代谢

reproductive [ˌriːprə'dʌktɪv] adj. 生殖的

hormone ['hɔːməʊn] n. 激素

bloodstream ['blʌdstriːm] n. 血流

secrete [sɪ'kriːt] vt. 分泌

infection [ɪn'fekʃən] n. 感染

vessel ['vesəl] n. 血管

lymph [lɪmf] n. 淋巴

protein ['prəʊtiːn] n. 蛋白质

molecule ['mɒlɪkjuːl] n. 分子

*Note*

glucose ['glu:kəʊs] n. 葡萄糖

urea [jʊ'ri:ə] n. 尿素

ribcage ['rɪbkeɪdʒ] n. 胸腔

**Task 5  Fill in the blanks with the words given below and change the word forms if necessary.**

1. Hawthorn is also recommended in cases of _____(function) heart pain and mild arrhythmias.

2. Potassium has an important role in the _____(regulate) of acid base balance.

3. The plants _____(growth) best in cool and damp conditions.

4. The discovery has promoted the research in human _____(reproductive).

5. _____(nervous) are long thin fibres that transmit messages between the brain and other parts of the body.

6. She apologized for the intrusion but said she had an urgent _____(messenger).

7. Insufficient sleep affects growth hormone _____(secrete) that is linked to obesity.

8. Antibiotics are _____(extensive) used in the patients suffered with viral encephalitis.

9. Those suffering from _____(infection) diseases were separated from the other patients.

10. Surrounded by famous mountains and great rivers, the city is rich in tourist resources because of its unique geographical _____(locate).

**Task 6  Choose the correct answer according to the passage.**

1. Which of the following statements is NOT the main function of the endocrine system? _____

A. regulating mood

B. regulating growth and development

C. regulating sexual function and reproductive processes

D. regulating body movement

2. What is the endocrine system in charge of? _____

A. breathing        B. cell growth        C. blood circulation    D. speaking

3. Which of the following statements is NOT true about hormones? _____

A. Hormones are parts of the foundation of the endocrine system

B. Hormones transfer information and instructions from one set of cells to another

C. One type of hormone is able to affect various types of cells

D. Hormones move through the bloodstream

4. What is lymph? _____

A. It's a clear and watery fluid containing proteins, salts, glucose, urea, and other substances

B. It's an extensive drainage network

C. It's an organ

D. It's a type of hormone

5. What is the function of the spleen? _____

A. It helps keep bodily fluid levels in balance and defends the body against infections

B. It protects the body, clearing worn-out red blood cells and other foreign bodies from the bloodstream to help fight off infection

*Note*

C. It selects and removes materials from the blood, processes them, and secretes the finished chemical products for use somewhere in the body

D. It regulates mood, growth and development, tissue function, metabolism, and sexual function and reproductive processes

**Task 7** **Arrange the following steps about first aid in proper sequence based on the medical procedure.**

_____ Take the casualty to hospital.

_____ Raise the injured hand of the casualty to control bleeding and apply a dressing.

_____ Place the casualty's hand in soft padding and in an elevation sling and a broad-fold bandage.

## New Words

padding ['pædɪŋ] n. 衬垫

elevation [ˌelɪ'veɪʃən] n. 高处,高地,高度

sling [slɪŋ] n. 悬带

**Passage B**

### Diabetes in China and Tips for Prevention

China's economic growth in the last several decades has dramatically transformed the nation's economic landscape, removing 500 million people from poverty. This progress, however, has been accompanied by an increase in some diseases, such as diabetes, notably associated with increased urbanization and changed lifestyles. Twenty-five years ago, the number of people with diabetes in China accounted for less than one percent. Today, China has more than 114 million people suffering from diabetes, the highest number of any country in the world.

It is estimated that 11. 6 percent of Chinese adults have diabetes, a proportion higher than the U. S. with 11. 3 percent. Experts blamed the increase in sedentary lifestyles, high consumption of sugary and high-calorie Western diets, excessive smoking and lack of exercise. According to some experts, India and China will have an increase of an additional 48. 5 million people with diabetes between 2007 and 2025.

Of the two kinds of diabetes, type 1 diabetes is diagnosed primarily in children and young adults, and has probably genetic and environmental components. Type 2 diabetes, which probably also has a small genetic component, is mostly caused by unhealthy lifestyles and obesity. Type 1 diabetes accounts for approximately 5 percent of all cases.

When it comes to type 2 diabetes, the most common type of diabetes, prevention is a big deal. It's especially important to make diabetes prevention a priority if you're at increased risk of diabetes, such as you're overweight or you have a family history of diabetes.

### 1. Get more physical activity

There are many benefits of regular physical activity. Exercise can help you lose weight, lower blood sugar, and boost sensitivity to insulin, which helps keep your blood sugar within a normal range.

Research shows that aerobic exercise and resistance training can help control diabetes. The greatest benefit comes from a fitness program that includes both.

*Note*

扫码听
课文 B

**2. Get plenty of fiber**

It's rough and tough. It may help you reduce risk of diabetes by improving blood sugar control, lower risk of heart disease, promote weight loss by helping you feel full.

Foods high in fiber include fruits, vegetables, beans, whole grains and nuts.

**3. Go for whole grains**

It's not clear why, but whole grains may reduce the risk of diabetes and help maintain blood sugar levels. Try to make at least half your grains whole grains. Many foods made from whole grains come ready to eat, including various breads, pasta products and cereals. Look for the word "whole" on the package and among the first few items in the ingredient list.

**4. Lose extra weight**

If you're overweight, diabetes prevention may hinge on weight loss. Every pound you lose can improve your health, and you may be surprised by how much. Participants in a large study who lost a modest amount of weight(around 7 percent of initial body weight) and exercised regularly reduced the risk of developing diabetes by almost 60 percent.

**5. Skip fad diets and just make healthier choices**

Low-carb diets, the glycemic index diet or other fad diets may help you lose weight at first. But their effectiveness at preventing diabetes isn't known, nor are their long-term effects. And by excluding or strictly limiting a particular food group, you may be giving up essential nutrients. Instead, make variety and portion control part of your healthy-eating plan.

## New Words & Phrases

diabetes [ˌdaɪəˈbiːtiːz] n. 糖尿病

sedentary [ˈsedəntərɪ] adj. 久坐的

sugary [ˈʃʊɡərɪ] adj. 含糖的

high-calorie [haɪ ˈkælərɪ] adj. 高热量的

diagnose [ˈdaɪəɡnəʊz] v. 诊断

primarily [ˈpraɪmərəlɪ] adv. 主要地

genetic [dʒɪˈnetɪk] adj. 遗传的，基因的

obesity [əʊˈbiːsətɪ] n. 肥胖

sensitivity [ˌsensɪˈtɪvətɪ] n. 敏感性

insulin [ˈɪnsjʊlɪn] n. 胰岛素

aerobic [eəˈrəʊbɪk] adj. 需氧的

resistance [rɪˈzɪstəns] n. 抵抗

fiber [ˈfaɪbə(r)] n. 纤维

whole grain 全谷类

cereal [ˈsɪərɪəl] n. 谷类

low-carb(abbr. low carbohydrate) 低碳水化合物

glycemic [ɡlaɪˈsemɪk] adj. 血糖的

*Note*

49

## Exercises

**Task 8   Match the words or phrases with similar meaning in the two columns.**

| A | B |
|---|---|
| 1. dramatically | a. evaluate |
| 2. consumption | b. related to blood sugar |
| 3. primarily | c. remarkably |
| 4. associate | d. precedence |
| 5. estimate | e. relate |
| 6. proportion | f. expense |
| 7. priority | g. sustain |
| 8. boost | h. mainly |
| 9. maintain | i. promote |
| 10. glycemic | j. ratio |

**Task 9   Choose the right answer to fill in the blanks in the passage.**

Raleigh，a nurse at Johns Hopkins Hospital， __1__ taking her niece to a movie __2__ one of the characters was a nurse. "In the movie，the little girl is dying. It's a very sad situation and the nurse comes in and says to the family quite __3__ , 'You all need to go home, visiting hours are over.' And she walks out of the room." says Raleigh. "I was thinking to __4__ , 'Gosh, does my niece think that this is what really happens? All nurses are like this or this is how we act __5__ patients?' It just made me sad. It just embarrassed me in front of my niece."

Raleigh's co-worker at the hospital, Neysa Ernst, says nurse portrayals on television are not much __6__ . "There are 2.9 million nurses in the United States. There are 790,000 physicians. And yet when you watch the TV programs, you see the physicians __7__ all of the work that nurses normally do," says Ernst. "Nurses are the ones __8__ are doing the EKGs. Nurses are the people who are taking the patient back and forth to the tests, making sure that procedures are administered __9__ . I don't see that on television."

A group of nursing students founded *The Truth about Nursing* nine years ago to encourage the media to present a more __10__ portrayal of their profession.

1. A. reminds     B. recalls     C. reuses     D. reviews
2. A. which     B. in which     C. in that     D. who
3. A. patiently     B. quietly     C. abruptly     D. gently
4. A. her     B. herself     C. you     D. myself
5. A. towards     B. with     C. by     D. on
6. A. worse     B. bad     C. better     D. good
7. A. doing     B. is doing     C. done     D. being done
8. A. which     B. that     C. whose     D. where
9. A. mistakenly     B. noticeably     C. pleasantly     D. appropriately
10. A. realistic     B. beautiful     C. important     D. evident

# Part 4　Write and Learn

**Prescription**

**Direction：Read the following writing sample carefully. Design and finish an imitated writing task with similar style.**

In the United States, a doctor sometimes may dictate prescriptions to nurses through phone calls, and signs his/her name on them later. Such a prescription should include the doctor's name, the patient's name, the patient's address and age, the date of the prescription made, etc. The following sample is a prescription. Read it and learn the meaning of the abbreviations of Rx., Sig. and Disp.

【Sample】

> Name：Sue White　　　　Age：23　　　　Date：06/11/2009
>
> Address：2020 5<sup>th</sup> Street,Seattle
>
> Rx.：Throat lozenge × 100 mg/tab
>
> Sig.：Six tabs.daily
>
> Disp.：50 tabs
>
> Name of doctor：Williams Lang
>
> Signature：*Williams Lang*

【Assignment】

Jenny Duncun, 35 years old, lives on 36 25<sup>th</sup> Ave. , New York. She's got a cold and went to see the doctor on July 28<sup>th</sup>, 2009. As she's also got a sore throat and a fever. Kate Longley, the doctor, prescribed 8 tablets of aspirin, 0. 5 gram per tablet and 30 tablets of throat lozenge, 100 mg per tablet for her. The doctor told Jenny that she should take the aspirin 1 tablet each time, three times a day after meals, and the lozenge 1 tablet each time, six times a day.

Name：_____ Age：_____ Date：_____

Address：_____

Rx. :_____

Sig. :_____

Disp. :_____

Name of doctor：Kate Longley

Signature：_____

*Note*

# Part 5  Prefixes, Suffixes & Roots

## Endocrine System（内分泌系统）

| 汉语（英语） | 常 用 词 根 | 例 词 |
|---|---|---|
| 分泌（secretion） | crin(o)-；secret(o)- | endocrine 内分泌；secretive 分泌的 |
| 腺（gland） | aden(o)- | adenoma 腺瘤；adenomyosis 子宫腺肌病 |
| 垂体（pituitary） | pitui-；hypophys- | pituitary 垂体；hypopituitarism 垂体功能减退 hypophyseal 垂体的；pituicyte 垂体细胞 |
| 甲状腺（thyroid） | thyr(o)- | thyroiditis 甲状腺炎；thyroxine 甲状腺素；thyrotrophin 促甲状腺激素 |
| 肾上腺（adrenal） | adren(o)- | adrenalitis 肾上腺炎；adrenaline 肾上腺素 |
| 胸腺（thymus） | thym(o)- | thymosin 胸腺素；thymoma 胸腺瘤 |
| 葡萄糖（glucose） | gluc(o)- | glucagon 胰高血糖素；glucokinase 葡萄糖激酶 |
| 钙（calcium） | calc(i)- | calcification 钙化；cholecalciferol 胆钙化醇 |

**Task 10  Learn the prefixes, suffixes or roots in the table by heart and then choose the best answer to finish the exercises.**

1. The correct spelling form of the word "内分泌" is _____.

A. endocrine        B. intracrine        C. intercrine        D. introcrine

2. Fill in the blank with the combining part for the medical term "子宫腺肌病"：_____ - myosis.

A. crino        B. gland        C. adeno        D. utero

3. The Chinese explanation for the word "hypopituitarism" is _____.

A. 下丘脑促垂体    B. 垂体功能亢进    C. 下丘脑垂体    D. 垂体功能减退

4. The Chinese meaning for the word "adenoma" is _____.

A. 腺瘤        B. 腺癌        C. 腺素        D. 肾上腺素

5. The correct Chinese equivalent for the word "thymosin" is _____.

A. 胸腺瘤        B. 胸腺素        C. 胸腺生成素        D. 胸腺生成

6. Which version of Chinese is right for the term "adrenaline"? _____

A. 去甲肾上腺素    B. 肾上腺皮质激素    C. 肾上腺素    D. 类肾上腺素

7. The English word defined as the inflammation of the thyroid is _____.

A. thyroiditis        B. adrenalitis        C. gonaditis        D. thymitis

8. The word formation of "calc(i)-" means _____.

A. kalium        B. natrium        C. calcium        D. iodium

9. The definition of "thymoma" is _____.

A. any disease of thymus            B. tumor of thymus

C. enlargement of thymus            D. hypertrophy of thymus

10. Which term is equal to the English term "cholecalciferol" in the following choices? _____

A. 钙化        B. 高钙        C. 降钙素        D. 胆钙化醇

# Midterm Review

## I Listening

### Part 1

**Questions 1-5**

- You will hear five patients describing their pain to the nurse.
- Where does each patient have pain?
- For questions 1-5，mark the correct letter A-H on your answer sheet.
- You will hear each conversation twice.

1. Connolly
2. Jameson
3. Jack
4. Swift
5. Douglas

A. in the eye

B. in the tooth

C. in the leg

D. in the back

E. in the chest

F. in the hand

G. in the forehead

H. in the knee

扫码听
对话

### Part 2

**Questions 6-10**

扫码听
对话

- You will hear a conversation between Mrs. Samira(the patient) and Mike(the ward nurse).
- For questions 6-10，decide if each sentence is correct or incorrect.
- If it is correct，put a tick（√）in the box next to A for Yes. If it is not correct，put a tick（√）in the box next to B for No.
- You will hear the conversation twice.

6. Mrs. Samira is alert and oriented.  A ☐
   B ☐

7. Mrs. Samira feels hot now.  A ☐
   B ☐

8. The nurse gives a pillow to the patient.  A ☐
   B ☐

9. The nurse will take the observation for the patient.  A ☐

*Note*

B 　☑

10. The patient is in recovery.　　　　　　　　A 　☐

B 　☐

**Part 3**

**Questions 11-16**

• You will hear two nurses talking about Annabel's obs.

• Listen and complete questions.

• You will hear the conversation twice.

扫码听
对话

St. Florence Hospital

　　Observation Chart

Admission observations

Date：20/09/2020

Time：10.00 hours

Full name：Annabel Marriot

DOB：03/08/1983

Doctor：Howland

Hosp. No.：673122

| | | | |
|---|---|---|---|
| T：____11____ | | P：____12____ | |
| BP：____13____ | | RR：____14____ | |
| $O_2$ SATS：____15____ | | Wt：____16____ | |

## Ⅱ Reading and Writing

**Part 1**

• Read the following passage.

• Choose the best word for each space.

**Fresh Sample**

It began as a typical working day. As a registered nurse, I traveled to clients' homes to complete paramedical health assessments 1. _____ an insurance company.

As I entered this lady's neat and attractive home, I smelled the delicious aroma of pies 2. _____. "Umm, sure smells good in here," I commented.

"I just put a couple of lemon meringue pies 3. _____ the oven. They're my husband's favorite," my client volunteered.

Returning to the purpose of my visit, we 4. _____ the questionnaire quickly. The last section involved collecting a urine sample.

"I collected it earlier 5. _____ saved it in the refrigerator," she said. "I'll get it for you."

6. _____ I emptied the sample into the collection tubes, I noticed the unusual thickness of it. When I tested it with a dip stick, I was 7. _____ at the extremely high protein content.

"Are you sure this is your urine sample?" I questioned. "8. _____ almost resembles egg whites."

"Yes, I distinctly remember placing it in the refrigerator in the bottom right-hand corner. Oh! Oh, no!" She wailed. "I've made a terrible mistake. Don't use that. I'll 9. _____ you a fresh

Note

sample. "

Not wishing to further embarrass the lady, I asked no more questions. But as I opened the door to leave her home, I 10. _____ her removing pies from the oven and the grinding sound of the garbage disposal.

No lemon meringue pie that night!

1. A. at
   B. for
   C. on
2. A. baking
   B. baked
   C. bakes
3. A. in
   B. with
   C. at
4. A. made
   B. collected
   C. completed
5. A. but
   B. and
   C. or
6. A. As
   B. Because
   C. If
7. A. mad
   B. shocked
   C. unhappy
8. A. This
   B. These
   C. It
9. A. bring
   B. send
   C. get
10. A. heard
    B. saw
    C. found

## Part 2

· Read the following passages.

· Choose the right answer which you think fits best according to the passages.

### First Aid

Doctors in hospital emergency rooms often see accidental poisoning patients. A frightened parent arrives with a child who swallowed a cleaning liquid, or perhaps the harmful substance is a medicine, or it might be a product meant to kill insects. These are common causes of accidental poisoning.

In cases like these, seek medical help as soon as possible. Save container of whatever causes the poisoning. And look on that container for information about anything that stops the effects of the poison. Save anything expelled from the mouth of the victim. That way, doctors can examine it.

In the past, some people forced poisoning victims to empty their stomachs. They used a liquid— syrup of ipecac—to do this. But a leading medical organization no longer advises parents to keep syrup of ipecac. The American Academy of Pediatrics says some poisons may cause additional damage when they come back up the throat.

Millions of people know how to give abdominal thrusts to save a person from choking on something trapped in the throat. The American Red Cross says a rescuer should first hit the person on the back between the shoulder bones five times. These back blows may ease the choking. If the airway is still blocked, the Red Cross suggests pushing five times hard along the victim's abdomen. The abdomen is the area between the chest and the hipbones. You can do these abdominal thrusts by getting directly behind a sitting or standing person. Put your arms around the victim's waist. Close one hand to form a ball. Place it over the upper part of the stomach, below the ribs. Place the other hand on top. Then push forcefully inward and upward. Repeat the abdominal thrusts until the object is expelled from the mouth. For someone in late pregnancy or who is very fat, place your hands higher than with normal abdominal thrusts. Place your hands at the base of the breastbone, just above the place where the lowest ribs join. Then begin pushing, as with the other victims.

The American Heart Association suggests another method for the same problem. The group advises chest thrusts instead of abdominal thrusts. For chest thrusts, put your arms under the victim's arms and your hands on the center of the victim's chest.

*Note*

55

Even if you are the person choking, you can still help yourself. Place a closed hand over the middle of your abdomen just above your waist. Take hold of that hand with your other hand. Find a hard surface like a chair and rest your body on it. Then push your closed hand in and up.

1. Which of the followings is not the common cause of accidental poisoning? _____

A. product meant to kill insects

B. medicine

C. pure water

2. What can you do when there is an accidental poisoning patient? _____

A. use syrup of ipecac to empty the stomach

B. save something expelled from the victim

C. hit the person on the back

3. The American Red Cross suggests that _____ if a person is choking.

A. hit the patient's back between the shoulder bones five times

B. wait for the medical help

C. use the syrup of ipecac to empty the stomach

4. If you are choking, you can _____.

A. hit your back by yourself

B. place your hand over the middle of the abdomen

C. ask for help

5. What's the main idea of the passage? _____

A. how to save the accidental poisoning patients

B. how to save the patients choking on something

C. some first aid skills

## Asthma

Asthma is a chronic breathing disorder characterized by repeating attacks of breathlessness. Some causes are common to the people with asthma, and some are more personal. Although the main causes of asthma are not fully understood, the most dangerous factor for developing asthma is inhaled asthma trigger. The triggers include house dust mites on bed, carpets furniture, pollution and pet, pollens, tobacco smoke and chemicals in the workplace.

For some people, asthma can even be triggered by certain medications, such as aspirin, and beta-blocks (which are used to treat high blood pressure, heart conditions and migraine). Other triggers include cold air, extreme emotional change such as anger or fear, and physical exercise. Regular physical activity is good for people with asthma, but it can also cause symptoms either during or right after being active.

The good news is that if you have good control of asthma, exercises should not be a problem for you. In fact, most people with asthma should be able to take part in any physical activities they like without causing asthma symptoms. Your healthcare provider may suggest an inhaler for about 15 minutes before exercise. This usually can prevent and control exercise-caused asthma.

6. The causes of asthma are the same for all people. _____

A. right          B. wrong          C. not mentioned

7. Extreme emotional change does no harm to people with asthma. _____

A. right          B. wrong          C. not mentioned

8. Although asthma cannot be cured, appropriate management can control the disorder and enable

people to enjoy good quality of life. _____

    A. right                 B. wrong                 C. not mentioned

9. Extreme emotional change won't cause any symptoms for people with asthma. _____

    A. right                 B. wrong                 C. not mentioned

10. Using an inhaler for about 15 minutes before exercise usually can prevent and control exercise-caused asthma. _____

    A. right                 B. wrong                 C. not mentioned

**Part 3**

    • Read the following conversation, and then filling the blanks with proper words.

    Helena: All right, Mylene. Let's get the next IV bag ready. Before we start, we need to wash our hands.

    Mylene: Oh, right. Of course.

    Helena: OK, now we can start. First, we'll check the IV solution against the IV prescription.

    Mylene: OK. The prescription is 5% dextrose.

    Helena: That's it. Here is the IV infusion. Can you check it with me? This is a bag of 5% dextrose.

    Mylene: Yes, I can see the label, 5% dextrose.

    Helena: Next, I'm going to prime the line. To prime the line, you run the IV fluid through the IV tubing of the giving set.

    Mylene: The giving set has one end to go into the IV bag and the other end is for connection to the patient's cannula. Is that right?

    Helena: That's right. We are going to run this IV infusion through an IV infusion pump. Next we need to set the rate on the infusion pump. What's the rate, Mylene?

    Mylene: The rate is 125 milliliters per hour.

    Helena: That's right. It's an 8-hour litre. After that, I'll start the infusion pump. Don't worry, Mr Lenworth, the pump is just running a test.

    Mylene: Oh, right. Noisy. Isn't it?

    Helena: Yes, it is. OK, that's ready. Now, I'll connect the IV to Mr. Lenworth's cannula. Then, I'll start the infusion pump. All right, Mr. Lenworth?

    Lenworth: Yes, that's fine.

    Helena: Now we both have to sign the IV prescription.

    Mylene: OK, here?

    Helena: That's right. The last thing is to write up the fluid balance chart.

    Mylene: OK, I think I have all that.

    Helena: Let's go over it again. Can you tell me the seven steps we went through?

    Mylene: Yes, I think I can. Before you start, wash your hands. First, check the IV bag against the IV order. Next, prime the line of the giving set. Then, set the rate on the infusion pump. After that, connect the IV to the patient's cannula and then start the infusion pump. Finally, sign the IV prescription and write up the IV infusion on the fluid balance chart.

    Helena: Well done.

We need to 1. _____ our hands.

We'll 2. _____ the IV solution against the IV prescription.

*Note*

I'm going to 3. _____ the line.

4. _____ the rate on the infusion pump.

I'll 5. _____ the IV to Mr. Lenworth's cannula.

I'll 6. _____ the infusion pump.

To 7. _____ the IV prescription.

To 8. _____ the fluid balance chart.

**Part 4**

Writing

• Read the discharge summary below.

• Use the information in the summary to write a report of no less than 100 words.

**Discharge Summary**

| Patient | Tom Smith | **Sex** | Male | **Age** | 15 |
| --- | --- | --- | --- | --- | --- |
| **Hospital day** | 10 days | | | | |
| **Date of admission** | May 15<sup>th</sup>, 2020 | | | | |
| **Condition on admission** | High fever, dry cough, no appetite | | | | |
| **Admission diagnosis** | Pneumonia | | | | |
| **Treatments** | Erythromycin to dephlogisticate | | | | |
| **Prognosis** | Improved, showing general state of health, had good appetite, stable condition | | | | |
| **Discharge instruction** | No medication, follow-up in one week with Dr. John | | | | |

*Note*

58

# Unit 6　The Immune System

## Learning Objectives：

To remember some key English words related to the immune system.

To understand the conversation about preoperative nursing and talk about the topic.

To read and understand the main ideas and the details of the passages about the immune system.

To learn to write a discharge summary with the help of the given sample writing.

To learn by heart some word roots，prefixes and suffixes about orientation system.

## Part 1　Look and Learn

**Warming-up 1：Look at the following picture，talk about them and then finish Task 1.**

IMMUNE SYSTEM

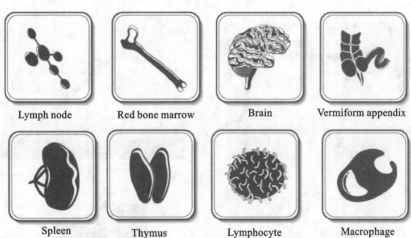

Lymph node　　　Red bone marrow　　　Brain　　　Vermiform appendix

Spleen　　　Thymus　　　Lymphocyte　　　Macrophage

## New Words

lymph [lɪmf] n. 淋巴

node [nəʊd] n. 节，结

marrow ['mærəʊ] n. 骨髓

appendix [ə'pendɪks] n. 阑尾

spleen [spliːn] n. 脾

thymus ['θaɪməs] n. 胸腺

*Note*

lymphocyte [ˈlɪmfəʊsaɪt] n. 淋巴细胞

macrophage [ˈmækrəʊfeɪdʒ] n. 巨噬细胞

**Task 1　Match the words in the left column with the explanations in the right column.**

| | |
|---|---|
| 1. antigen | A. a harmful substance; a disease-causing agent like a bacteria, virus, or parasite |
| 2. antibody | B. a foreign substance that enters the body and stimulates the body to produce antibodies against it; it triggers a response from the immune system |
| 3. pathogen | C. a rise of body temperature above the normal, caused by the response to an infection |
| 4. fever | D. blood cells that engulf and digest bacteria and fungi |
| 5. leukocyte | E. a protein produced by blood plasma that fights pathogens |

**Warming-up 2：Look at the following pictures about medical instruments, talk about them and then finish Task 2.**

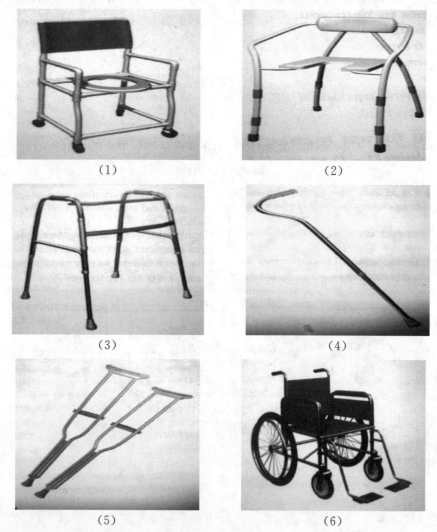

(1)　　　　　　　　　(2)

(3)　　　　　　　　　(4)

(5)　　　　　　　　　(6)

## New Words

commode [kəˈməʊd] n. 洗脸台，便桶

crutch [krʌtʃ] n. 拐杖

**Task 2   Label the pictures above using the words below.**

shower chair(沐浴椅)                    walking frame(助行架)

crutches(拐杖)                           walking stick(手杖)

wheelchair（轮椅）                       commode chair(流动座便椅)

(1) _____

(2) _____

(3) _____

(4) _____

(5) _____

(6) _____

# Part 2   Listen and Learn

## Situation Dialogue：Preoperative Nursing

**Task 3   Listen to the audio episode one and fill in the missing words referring to the original text. Then check your writing against the original.**

Nurse：Morning, Mr. Peter. I am Cathy. Did you sleep well last night?

Patient：Morning, Cathy. I was a little nervous about the 1. _____, so I didn't sleep that well.

Nurse：Yes, it's hard for everyone at this point. Do you have any questions about the surgery?

Patient：Mm, I signed the consent form two days ago, and I saw the 2. _____ of the operation in the form, such as the complications from the 3. _____, the 4. _____, and even death. I am a little afraid of these things.

Nurse (smiles and touches the patient's hand)：I understand it's not easy for you. Actually the consent form tells us all kinds of the possibilities during the surgery, but these risks are very small and not likely to happen to you. It's just 5. _____ hospital procedure.

Patient：I see. I hope my surgery is successful. Especially my child is only five years old.

Nurse (smiles)：It will be fine. You should trust the doctors. And you have been on a 6. _____ diet for three days, right?

Patient：Yes. May I eat today?

Nurse：Yes, but only clear 7. _____ for today. Then you'll start NPO after midnight.

**Task 4   Listen to the audio episode two and complete the answers according to the questions.**

1. When will the patient be given an enema?

The patient should be given an enema tonight 1. _____.

2. Why will the patient be given an enema?

The enema causes the patient to have a 2. _____ and then lower the risk of contamination from the bowel content.

3. What are two more things before the surgery?

Tomorrow morning the patient will be given a nasogastric tube to keep the 3. _____

扫码听
对话 1

扫码听
对话 2

*Note*

61

empty. And the patient will keep tube for a few days for gastric decompression.

# Part 3　Read and Learn

扫码听
课文 A

**Passage A**

### Coping with Rare Genetic Diseases in China

With a population of 1.4 billion, China shares the largest amount of rare genetic diseases worldwide. Current estimates suggest that there are over ten million individuals afflicted with chromosomal diseases and well over one million individuals with monogenic diseases.

Genetic diseases, categorized as chromosomal diseases and monogenic diseases, affect approximately 1% of all individuals globally. There are over 100 different recognized chromosomal diseases. Chromosomal diseases are believed to be caused in the early period of human development. The most prevalent is Down syndrome (DS) with an incidence of 1 in 700 births.

Care of patients with rare genetic diseases remains a largely unmet need due to the paucity of available and affordable treatments. Over recent years, there is an increasing recognition of the need for affirmative action by government, health providers, clinicians and patients.

The advent of new next generation sequencing (NGS) technologies, such as whole genome sequencing, offers a new opportunity to provide large-scale population screening of the Chinese population to identify the molecular causes of rare genetic diseases. As a replacement for lack of effective treatments, recent development and implementation of noninvasive prenatal testing (NIPT) in China has the greatest potential, as a single technology, for reducing the number of children born with rare genetic diseases.

Even though the number of patients with genetic disease in China is very high, most stay confined in the home and do not participate in daily life. Except in special events dedicated to a particular disease or disability, patients with genetic diseases are rarely seen in public. As in many other cultures, traditional Chinese values discourage a family from allowing the affected individual to go out. Without understanding the causes of the diseases, the society in the past tended to blame the family for the disability. Also, within the family, when a child was born with a genetic disease, there was a strong tendency for one of the parents to blame the other for bringing disrepute to the family, causing shame and guilt.

There is a cultural shift in the way families are coping with genetic diseases in China. Now, more than ever, families and patients are presenting to clinics to seek the medical opinion of doctors regarding the diseases and possible treatments to alleviate suffering. Medical doctors have become increasingly skilled at making the correct clinical diagnosis for most genetic diseases and some patients are willing to pay a small DNA testing fee to define the causative familial mutations. This is an important step if members of the families have married and are planning to have children, enabling the option of prenatal diagnosis.

Once parents have a better understanding of their child's disease and potential treatments, they are finding it much easier to come to terms with the disease in the family and cope better with the day to day impact of the disease burden.

*Note*

**Task 5  Fill in the blanks with the words given below and change the word forms if necessary.**

1. In light of the COVID-19 pandemic, experts are training their sights on how AI can help improve the public health system through enhanced epidemic research, _____ (gene) testing and drug development.

2. Rub the cream into the _____ (affect) areas.

3. We have to protect the health of our health _____ (provide) who are fighting against the COVID-19 virus.

4. All those with a fever should voluntarily go to fever _____ (clinician) for treatment, where they can have free nucleic acid and antibody tests for the virus.

5. Lung cancer _____ (screen) is recommended for older adults who are longtime smokers and who don't have any signs or symptoms of lung cancer.

6. Jinhua Qinggan Granule and Lianhua Qingwen Capsule/Granule have proven to be effective in the _____ (treat) of mild COVID-19 cases.

7. The number of registered volunteers reached 169 million by the end of last year on the Chinese mainland, who assisted in health, education, poverty alleviation, eldercare, environment, _____ (disable), culture and sports, among other areas.

8. The hospice aims to ease the _____ (suffer) of the dying.

9. A 68-year-old woman in Jingzhou, Hubei province tested positive for the novel coronavirus and _____ (diagnosis) with the disease on Feb. 8th.

10. _____ (potential) risk factors were evaluated, such as family history, nutrition, exercise, smoking status, and alcohol consumption.

**Task 6  Choose the correct answer according to the passage.**

1. What's the total number of people with genetic diseases estimated in China? _____
A. 10,000,000                          B. 100,000
C. About more than 10,100,000          D. 1.4 billion

2. What is the best replacement of the phrase "afflicted with" in the first paragraph? _____
A. diagnosed by      B. suffering from      C. presented with      D. tested out

3. Which of the following statements is true about genetic diseases? _____
A. Both chromosomal and monogenic diseases are genetic diseases
B. There are only 100 different chromosomal diseases
C. Chromosomal diseases are believed to be caused throughout human development
D. 1 from 700 cases of Down syndrome (DS) can be cured

4. Which of the following statements is an NGS technology? _____
A. ultrasound                          B. pregnancy hypertension test
C. NIPT                                D. hepatitis B test

5. How do Chinese families cope with genetic diseases now? _____
A. The patients stay home to avoid being seen in public
B. They seek medical opinions and possible treatments from skilled doctors
C. They blame each other in the family for disability
D. They refuse to pay for DNA testing fee for prenatal diagnosis because it's not worth it

*Note*

**Task 7   Arrange the following steps in proper sequence based on the medical procedures.**

**Recovery Position**

_____ Turn the casualty's head towards you and tilt it back slightly to open the airway.

_____ Readjust the casualty's head so that it is now well back to make sure the airway stays open.

_____ Place the arm nearest you by the casualty's side. Keeping his hand flat, slide it well under his buttock.

_____ Kneel beside the casualty. About 22.5 cm from his chest and support his head with one hand. Grasp the casualty's clothes at the hip farthest from you and pull him towards you until he is resting against your knees.

_____ Slightly raise the farthest leg at the heel, bring it towards you and cross it over his other leg. Then bring the casualty's other arm up and lay it across his chest with the hand, pointing towards his opposite shoulder.

_____ Working on the uppermost limbs, bond first the arm, and then the leg into a convenient position to prevent the casualty rolling on to his face.

_____ The arm behind the casualty should now be free. If it is not, carefully case it out from under his back and leave it lying parallel to his body to prevent him rolling on to his back.

## New Words

tilt [tɪlt] v. 使倾斜

buttock ['bʌtək] n. 臀部，屁股

bond [bɒnd] v. 使结合

parallel ['pærəlel] adj. 平行的

**Passage B**

扫码听
课文 B

### AIDS

People have been warned about HIV and AIDS for over twenty years now. AIDS has already killed millions of people. AIDS is one of the bigger problems facing the world today and nobody is beyond its reach. Everyone should know the basic facts about AIDS. AIDS stands for acquired immunodeficiency (or immune deficiency) syndrome. It results from infection with a virus called HIV, which stands for human immunodeficiency virus. This disease primarily spread through sexual intercourse and blood. This virus infects key cells in the human body called CD4-positive (CD4$^+$) T cells. These cells are part of the body's immune system, which fights infections and various cancers.

**The latest statistics on the world epidemic of AIDS & HIV at the end of 2007**

| | | |
|---|---|---|
| People living with HIV/AIDS | total | 33,200,000 (30,600,000-36,100,000) |
| | adults | 30,800,000 (28,200,000-33,600,000) |
| | women | 15,400,000 ( 13,900,000-16,600,000) |
| | children (≤15 years old) | 2,500,000 (2,200,000-2,600,000) |
| People newly infected with HIV/AIDS | total | 2,500,000 (1,800,000-4,100,000) |
| | adults | 2,100,000 (1,400,000-3,600,000) |
| | children (≤15 years old) | 420,000(350,000-540,000) |

续表

| Death toll of HIV infection | total | 2,100,000 (1,900,000-2,400,000) |
|---|---|---|
| | adults | 1,700,000 (1,600,000-2,100,000) |
| | children (≤15 years old) | 330,000 (310,000-380,000) |

Because the internal organs where opportunistic infections occur and the sites where tumors arise are different, symptoms are complex and varied.

Commonly seen symptoms are as follows:

• General symptoms: persistent fever, weakness, night sweats, superficial lymphadenopathy, weight loss.

• Respiratory symptoms: long-term cough, chest pain, difficulty breathing, blood in sputum (severe cases).

• Gastrointestinal symptoms: anorexia, nausea, vomiting, diarrhea, blood in the stool (severe cases).

• Nervous system symptoms: dizziness, headache, unresponsiveness, mental decline, mental disorders, seizures, hemiplegia, dementia.

• Skin and mucous membrane symptoms: herpes simplex, herpes zoster, oral and pharyngeal mucosa inflammation and ulceration.

In addition, a variety of malignant tumors can occur. Kaposi's sarcoma can be seen with red or purple macules, papules, and infiltrating masses found on the skin.

Clearly, the symptoms of AIDS are very complex.

The diagnosis of HIV infection can be made by detecting the presence of disease-fighting proteins called antibodies in the blood. Two different types of antibody tests, enzyme-linked immunoassay (ELISA) and Western blot, are available.

You can decrease your chances of being infected with HIV by avoiding high-risk behaviors.

◆ Abstain from unsafe sex, or have sex with only one partner who is also committed to having sex with only you.

◆ Use condoms with each act of sexual intercourse.

◆ If you use intravenous drugs, never share needles.

◆ If you are a health care worker, strictly follow universal precautions (the established infection-control procedures to avoid contact with bodily fluids).

◆ If you are a woman thinking about becoming pregnant, have a test for HIV beforehand, especially if you have a history of behaviors that put you at risk of HIV infection. Pregnant women who are HIV-positive need special prenatal care and medications to decrease the risk that HIV will pass to their newborn babies.

The prevention and treatment for people with HIV has improved enormously since the mid-1990s, but there is still no way to cure AIDS. The general principle of the treatment included anti-infection, anti-tumor, eliminating or restraint the HIV and enhancement organism immunity function.

## New Words

anorexia [ˌænəˈreksɪə] n. 食欲减退，厌食

condom [ˈkɒndɒm] n. 避孕套

dementia [dɪˈmenʃə] n. 痴呆

diarrhea [ˌdaɪə'rɪə] n. 痢疾，腹泻

hemiplegia [ˌhemɪ'pliːdʒɪə] n. 偏瘫，半身麻痹，半身不遂

herpes ['hɜːpiːz] n. 疱疹

immunoassay [ˌɪmjʊnəʊ'æseɪ] n. 免疫测定

lymphadenopathy ['lɪmˌfædɪ'nɒpəθɪ] n. 淋巴结病

macula ['mækjʊlə] n. 斑点，污点，黑点，斑疹

malignant [mə'lɪgnənt] adj. 恶性的

prenatal [ˌpriː'neɪtəl] adj. 出生以前的

ulceration [ˌʌlsə'reɪʃən] n. 溃疡

zoster ['zɒstə(r)] n. 带状疱疹

## Exercises

**Task 8　Match the words or phrases with similar meaning in the two columns.**

| A | B |
|---|---|
| 1. immature | a. being on or near the surface |
| 2. anorexia | b. existing or occurring before birth |
| 3. anemia | c. feeling of sickness or disgust |
| 4. superficial | d. physical or mental weariness resulting from exertion |
| 5. nausea | e. paralysis affecting only one side of the body |
| 6. hemiplegia | f. condition of the blood caused by a lack of red corpuscles |
| 7. prenatal | g. loss of appetite, especially as a result of disease |
| 8. macula | h. of or relating to circulatory system |
| 9. fatigue | i. not fully grown or developed |
| 10. circulatory | j. a spot, stain |

**Task 9　Choose the right answer to fill in the blanks in the passage.**

When it comes to hospital care, Jody Baker has a unique perspective—as both a caregiver and a patient.

Twenty-three years ago, Jody Baker, then 24, was on her way home from work when her life was changed forever. A catastrophic(悲惨的) car accident left her with multiple injuries, including ___1___ bones and a traumatic brain ___2___.

Taken to JFK Medical Center in Edison, Jody wasn't expected to live. She spent a month in the ___3___ care unit in a coma(昏迷). And while she doesn't recall the accident or much about her stay at JFK, she has no doubt that the great care she ___4___ there helped save her life.

Once stable enough to travel, Jody was ___5___ to Underwood-Memorial Hospital in Woodbury so she could continue her ___6___ closer to home. While at Underwood, she endured months of painful rehabilitation and ___7___ therapy.

"The nurses at Underwood were wonderfully caring and vigilant in ___8___ to the needs of this bedridden(卧床不起的), brain injured patient," said Jody.

But from tragedy came triumph. When Jody was finally able to return to work, she realized she wanted to do something meaningful with her second chance at life. Jody wanted to become a nurse.

She earned her associate's degree in Nursing from Gloucester County College. She has been working as the critical care clinical nurse ___9___ at a medical center and recently accepted a position as a registered nurse in CT angiography(血管造影法).

Jody feels the accident was meant to be. She believes that she has been ___10___ with the gift to help others who were also given a second chance at life. She's held hands with families as their loved ones were permitted to die with dignity, has calmed confused patients and supported those who thought there was no hope.

"What goes around comes around," said Jody. "Someday, I will be the patient again. I have no doubt that some wonderful nurse will be my guardian angel."

1. A. breaking      B. broke       C. broken       D. break
2. A. hurt          B. injury      C. damage       D. harm
3. A. extensive     B. intensive   C. inclusive    D. exclusive
4. A. took          B. accepted    C. adopted      D. received
5. A. transferred   B. changed     C. transmitted  D. moved
6. A. recover       B. recovery    C. covering     D. coverage
7. A. mental        B. radiation   C. drug         D. physical
8. A. meeting       B. serving     C. attending    D. satisfying
9. A. specialist    B. teacher     C. worker       D. staff
10. A. registered   B. admitted    C. assessed     D. blessed

## Part 4   Write and Learn

### Discharge Summary

**Direction:** Read the following writing sample carefully. Design and finish an imitated writing task with similar style.

出院小结

出院小结是患者住院诊疗经过的记录,便于以后复查时参考,也叫出院记录。出院小结内容包括患者基本信息、入院诊断、出院诊断、入院情况、检查体征、治疗情况、出院时恢复情况、复诊建议、用药建议和生活方式指导等。

【Sample】

| Patient: Zhang Jun | Sex: Male | Age: 18 |
|---|---|---|
| HOD (hospital day) | 6 days | |
| DOA (date of admission) | October 7th, 2008 | |
| Attending physician | Yu Bai | |
| Conditions on admission | Vomiting for unknown reason | |
| AD (admitting diagnosis) | Acute gastroenteritis | |
| Hospital course | The patient was admitted and placed on fluid rehydration and mineral supplement | |
| DOD (date of discharge) | October 12th, 2008 | |
| Conditions on discharge | The patient improved, showing gradual resolution of nausea and vomiting. The patient was discharged in stable condition | |

*Note*

续表

| DD (discharge diagnosis) | Acute gastroenteritis |
|---|---|
| Prognosis | Good. No medications needed after discharge. But if this patient can not get used to Chinese food, she had better return to UK as soon as possible to prevent the relapse（复发）of acute gastroenteritis |

The patient is to follow up with Dr. Yu Bai in one week. _____

Yu Bai　　　　D:12/10/2008

【Assignment】

**Direction：Read the information below and fill in the discharge summary.**

A patient's information：The patient was called Tom Smith, and he was 15 years old. He was admitted because of high fever, dry cough and no appetite on April 5, 2008. First, he was diagnosed as pneumonia and placed on erythromycin by attending physician Dr. John. After 15 days, the patient improved, showing general state of health. And the patient had good appetite. The patient was discharged in stable condition. At last, he was diagnosed as pneumonia, and Dr. John told the patient that no medications needed after discharge. The patient is to follow up with him in one week.

| Patient： | Sex： | Age： |
|---|---|---|
| HOD（hospital day） | | |
| DOA（date of admission） | | |
| Attending physician | | |
| Conditions on admission | | |
| AD（admitting diagnosis） | | |
| Hospital course | | |
| DOD（date of discharge） | | |
| Conditions on discharge | | |
| DD（discharge diagnosis） | | |
| Prognosis | | |

The patient is to follow up with Dr. John in one week. _____

John　　　　D:20/04/2008

# Part 5　Prefixes, Suffixes & Roots

## Orientation System（方位系统）

| 汉语（英语） | 常用词根 | 例　　　词 |
|---|---|---|
| 上（up） | epi-；<br>super-；<br>supra- | epicytoma 上皮瘤；superconductor 超导体；supraclavicular 锁骨上的；epinephrine 肾上腺素；epiderm（表皮） |

续表

| 汉语(英语) | 常用词根 | 例　词 |
|---|---|---|
| 下(down) | infer(o)-；infra-；sub-；hypo- | inferolateral 下侧的；infraorbital 眼眶下的；subaxillary 腋下的；subcutaneous（hypodermic）皮下的 |
| 左(left) | leva-；levo- | levamizole 左旋咪唑；levocardiogram 左侧心电图 |
| 右(right) | dextr(o)-；dexter- | dextrocardiogram 右侧心电图；dextrocular 惯用右眼的；dextrocardia（dexiocardia）右位心 |
| 前(front) | ante-；pre-；pro- | antenatal 产前的；preoperative 术前的；precordium 心前区；prostatic 前列腺的；prophylaxis 预防法 |
| 后(behind) | post-；retr(o)- | postpartum 产后的；postoperative 术后的；retrobulbar 眼球后的；retrobronchial 支气管后的 |
| 内(inside) | endo-；intra- | endocardium 心内膜；endocrine 内分泌的；intravenous 静脉内的；intramuscular 肌内的；intrauterine 子宫内的 |
| 外(outside) | ect(o)-；exo-；extra- | ectohormone 外激素；exocervix 外子宫颈；extraarticular 关节外的；extracorporeal 体外的；extracranial 颅外的 |
| 中心(center) | centro- | centrocyte 中心细胞；centrokinesis 中枢性运动 |
| 中间(middle) | medi(o)- | media 介质 |
| 周围(around) | circum-；peri- | circumcision 包皮环切术；periodontitis 牙周炎 |

**Task 10　Learn the prefixes, suffixes or roots in the table by heart and then choose the best answer to finish the exercises.**

1. The word meaning "of the area beneath the skin" is _____.

A. hypotension　　　　B. hypodermic　　　　C. hypothermia　　　　D. hypothyroid

2. On or of the outside is called _____.

A. extent　　　　B. extant　　　　C. extinct　　　　D. external

3. The equivalent to the word "endocardium" is the Chinese word _____.

A. 心内膜　　　　B. 内分泌　　　　C. 子宫颈内　　　　D. 囊内的

4. The correct spelling for the word "中枢性运动" is _____.

A. centriole　　　　B. centrocyte　　　　C. centrokinesis　　　　D. centroplasm

5. The English term for "眼球后的" is _____.

A. retrocecal　　　　B. retrobulbar　　　　C. retrobronchial　　　　D. retrocolic

6. What is the Chinese term for "levocardiogram"? _____

A. 左甲状腺素　　　　B. 左位心　　　　C. 左旋咪唑　　　　D. 左侧心电图

7. The English term for "肘前的" is _____.

A. antecubital　　　　B. antebrachial　　　　C. antecubita　　　　D. anteflexion

8. The Chinese term for "circumanal" is _____.

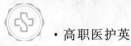

A. 阑尾周围的　　　　B. 包皮环切术　　　　C. 肛门周围的　　　　D. 眼周围的

9．The Chinese term for "dextrocular" is _____.

A. 右位心　　　　　　B. 惯用右眼的　　　　C. 右侧心电图　　　　D. 右旋

10．What is the Chinese term for "supracapsulin"? _____

A. 锁骨上的　　　　　B. 主动脉上的　　　　C. 视交叉上的　　　　D. 肾上腺素

# Unit 7　The Urinary System

## Learning Objectives:

To remember some key English words related to the urinary system.

To understand the conversation about postoperative nursing discussion and talk about the topic.

To read and understand the main ideas and the details of the passages about the urinary system.

To learn to write a recommendation letter with the help of the given sample writing.

To learn by heart some word roots, prefixes and suffixes about the urinary system.

## Part 1　Look and Learn

**Warming-up 1: Look at the following picture, talk about them and then finish Task 1.**

URINARY SYSTEM

Main vein to the heart carries cleaned blood

Main artery from heart brings blood with wastes

Right kidney

Left kidney

Ureter carries urine

Ureter

Nerve that tells brain the bladder is full

Bladder collects urine

Muscle to keep bladder closed

Urethra

Nerve that tells bladder to open

## New Words

kidney ['kɪdnɪ] n. 肾脏

Note

71

ureter [juˈriːtə(r)] n. 输尿管
bladder [ˈblædə(r)] n. 膀胱
nerve [nɜːv] n. 神经
muscle [ˈmʌsl] n. 肌肉
urethra [juˈriːθrə] n. 尿道

**Task 1　Match the words in the left column with the explanations in the right column.**

| 1. urethra | A. the canal that in most mammals conveys urine from the bladder out of the body |
| --- | --- |
| 2. ureter | B. the tube that conveys urine from the kidney to the urinary bladder or cloaca |
| 3. bladder | C. long thin fibres that transmit messages between your brain and other parts of your body |
| 4. nerve | D. a piece of tissue inside your body that connects two bones and which you use when you make a movement |
| 5. muscle | E. the part of your body where urine is stored until it leaves your body |

**Warming-up 2：Look at the following pictures about medical instruments, talk about them and then finish Task 2.**

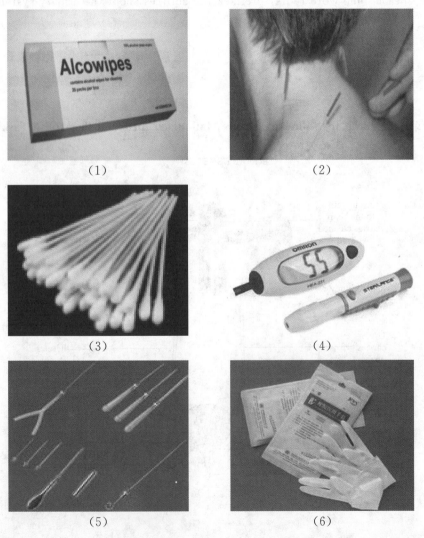

(1)　　　　　　　　　(2)

(3)　　　　　　　　　(4)

(5)　　　　　　　　　(6)

**New Words**

swab [swɒb] n. 拭子，药签

lancet ['lɑːnsɪt] n. 刺血针

acupuncture ['ækjʊˌpʌŋktʃə(r)] n. 针灸(疗法)

glucometer [glu:'kəʊ'mɪtə] n. 血糖仪

**Task 2　Match the picture number with the proper English and Chinese meaning.**

| Picture number | English | Chinese |
|---|---|---|
| | cotton swab | 棉签 |
| | alcohol wipe | 酒精棉 |
| | lancet | 刺血针 |
| | acupuncture | 针灸 |
| | medical rubber gloves | 医用橡胶手套 |
| | glucometer | 血糖仪 |

# Part 2　Listen and Learn

## Situation Dialogue：Postoperative Nursing Discussion

**Task 3　Listen to the audio episode one and fill in the missing words referring to the original text. Then check your writing against the original.**

Head nurse：Hello，everyone. Let's start with Mrs. John. Mrs. John is a 40-year-old American lady and was 1. _____ last Friday. From her biopsy she was diagnosed with rectum cancer 6 months ago in our hospital. A colostomy was performed on her at 10：00 am yesterday. She is fully awake and 2. _____ from the procedure. We are going to talk about her nursing implementation，especially the stoma care after the surgery.

Nurse 1：Mm，I examined her yesterday after she came back from the OR(operating rome). I feel that she's doing well. Her 3. _____ signs are good，except for a slight fever. But that's 4. _____ after the surgery. The stoma is swollen，but the 5. _____ around the stoma is good.

Nurse 2：Yes，we need to pay close attention to the stoma.

Head nurse：What kind of stoma is normal postoperation?

Nurse 1：Stoma is initially edematous and shrinks over the next 4 to 6 weeks. A normal stoma is moist and reddish pink. I think Mrs. John's stoma is a standard.

Head nurse：Any other signs? How about the skin?

扫码听
对话1

**Task 4　Listen to the audio episode two and complete the answers according to the questions.**

1. What's the first step of the pouching system?

The first step is to _____ our hands and apply _____ _____.

2. What should we do after the removal of the protective backing?

Apply _____ _____.

3. What should we do if the pouch is open?

Don't forget to _____ the end of pouch if it is open.

扫码听
对话2

*Note*

# Part 3  Read and Learn

扫码听
课文 A

**Passage A**

### Urinary Tract Infections

It was only 10:00 am, but Tracy had already visited the bathroom six times that morning. Sometimes she barely had time to ask the teacher for permission because the urge to pee was so intense. Did she drink too much orange juice for breakfast? Nope — although she really had to go, only a little urine came out each time. And every time she peed, she felt a burning sensation. What was going on?

Tracy's experience is not unusual. Her problem, a urinary tract infection, is one of the most common reasons that teens — especially girls — visit a doctor.

A bacterial urinary tract infection (UTI) is the most common kind of infection affecting the urinary tract. Urine, or pee, is the fluid that is filtered out of the bloodstream by the kidney. Urine contains salts and waste products, but it doesn't normally contain bacteria. When bacteria get into the bladder or the kidney and multiply in the urine, a UTI can result.

There are three main types of UTI. Bacteria that infect only the urethra (the short tube that delivers urine from the bladder to the outside of the body) cause urethritis.

Bacteria can also cause a bladder infection, which is called cystitis. Another, more serious, kind of UTI is infection of the kidney itself, known as pyelonephritis. With this type of UTI, a person often has back pain, high fever and vomiting.

The most common type of UTI, the bladder infection, causes mostly just discomfort and inconvenience. Bladder infections can be quickly and easily treated. And it's important to get treatment promptly to avoid the more serious infection that reaches the kidney. Remember that although urinary tract infections are uncomfortable and often painful, they are very common and easily treated. The sooner you contact your doctor, the sooner you'll be able to get rid of the problem.

## New Words

barely ['beəlɪ] adv. 几乎不

sensation [sen'seɪʃən] n. 感觉

urinary ['jʊərɪnərɪ] adj. 尿的,泌尿的

infection [ɪn'fekʃən] n. 感染,传染,传染病

pee [piː] v. 撒尿,小便
　　　　n. 撒尿,尿

filter ['fɪltə(r)] v. 过滤,渗透

bloodstream ['blʌdstriːm] n. 体内循环的血液

bacteria [bæk'tɪərɪə] n. (pl.) 细菌

urethritis [ˌjʊərɪ'θraɪtɪs] n. 尿道炎

cystitis [sɪs'taɪtɪs] n. 膀胱炎

pyelonephritis [ˌpaɪələʊne'fraɪtɪs] n. 肾盂肾炎

vomit ['vɒmɪt] v. 呕吐,(使)呕吐
　　　　n. 呕吐,呕吐物,催吐剂

*Note*

discomfort [dɪsˈkʌmfət] vt. 使……不舒服
n. 不适
promptly [ˈprɒmptlɪ] adv. 迅速地，立即地
painful [ˈpeɪnfʊl] adj. 痛苦的，疼痛的

**Task 5 Fill in the blanks with the words given below and change the word forms if necessary.**

1. Heartburn is described as a harsh, burning _____ (sense) in the area in between your ribs or just below your neck.

2. Worms move into blood vessels that supply the intestinal and _____ (urine) systems.

3. If light or sound _____ (filter) into a place, it comes in weakly or slowly, either through a partly covered opening, or from a long distance away.

4. During this time, he contracted _____ (urethra), an inflammation of the urethra that results in painful urination.

5. Interstitial _____ (cystic) is a chronic pain condition related to inflammation of the bladder. The cause is unknown.

6. Within a few days she had become seriously ill, suffering great pain and _____ (comfort).

7. But it means that we get ill less often and when we do get sick, we recover more _____ (prompt).

8. Her glands were swollen and _____ (pain).

9. The team says the _____ (bacteria) was changed so it cannot cause harm if it escapes.

10. Deaths from HIV _____ (infect) and AIDS raise a tremendous problem in Africa and other parts of the world.

**Task 6 Choose the correct answer according to the passage.**

1. Why did Tracy have to visit bathroom so often? _____
A. Because she drank too much juice
B. Because she didn't want to ask the teacher for permission.
C. Because she suffered from pyelonephritis.
D. Because she felt a burning sensation.

2. Which of the followings is not the main type of urinary tract infection? _____
A. urethritis        B. cystitis        C. pyelonephritis        D. prostatitis

3. According to the passage, a person who suffers from pyelonephritis may often have _____.
A. back pain        B. high fever        C. vomiting        D. all of the above

4. Which of the followings is the most common type of urinary tract infection? _____
A. cystitis        B. urethritis        C. pyelonephritis        D. nephritis

5. Which of the following statements is not true according to the passage? _____
A. Urine contains salts and waste products
B. When waste products get into the bladder or the kidney and multiply in the urine, a urinary tract infection can result
C. Getting treatment often can avoid the more serious infection that reaches the kidney
D. A person with cystitis often has back pain, high fever and vomiting

**Task 7   Arrange the following steps in proper sequence based on the medical procedure.**

_____ Apply pressure to the wound: Remove or cut casualty's clothing to expose wound. Apply direct pressure over wound. Cover wound with sterile dressing. Apply a pad.

_____ Bandage wound: Bandage firmly in place. Apply another dressing or pad if bleeding continues.

_____ Raise and support injured part: Lie casualty down. Raise injured part above level of heart. Handle gently if you suspect a fracture.

_____ Check circulation below wound.

_____ Wait for an ambulance if severe bleeding persists.

## New Words

扫码听
课文 B

expose [ɪk'spəʊz] v. 使暴露

sterile ['steraɪl] adj. 无菌的

fracture ['fræktʃə(r)] n. 骨折

circulation [ˌsɜːkjʊ'leɪʃən] n. 血液循环

persist [pə'sɪst] v. 坚持，继续存在

**Passage B**

**Acute Kidney Failure**

Acute kidney failure is the sudden loss of your kidneys' ability to perform their main function — eliminate excess fluid and waste material from your blood. When your kidneys lose their filtering ability, dangerous levels of fluid and waste accumulate in your body.

Acute kidney failure is the most common in people who are already hospitalized, particularly people who need intensive care. Acute kidney failure tends to occur after complicated surgery, after a severe injury or when blood flow to your kidneys is disrupted.

Loss of kidney function may also develop gradually over time, with few signs or symptoms in the early stages. In this case, it's referred to as chronic kidney failure. High blood pressure and diabetes are the most common causes of chronic kidney failure.

Acute kidney failure can be serious and generally requires intensive treatment. Unlike the chronic form, however, acute kidney failure is reversible and if you're otherwise in good health you should recover normal kidney function within a few weeks. If acute kidney failure occurs in the context of severe chronic illness — a heart attack, stroke, overwhelming infection — the outcome is often worse.

Signs and symptoms of acute kidney failure may include the followings.

• Decreased urine output, although occasionally urine output remains normal.

• Fluid retention, causing swelling in your legs, ankles or feet.

• Drowsiness.

• Shortness of breath.

• Fatigue.

• Confusion.

• Seizures or coma in severe cases.

• Chest pain related to pericarditis, an inflammation of the sac-like membrane that envelops your heart...

Some people don't notice any early signs or symptoms, but are more bothered by the underlying problems causing the sudden kidney failure.

*Note*

Your kidneys are two bean-shaped organs, each about the size of your fist. They're located at the back of your upper abdomen, one on either side of your spine. Your kidneys are part of a system that removes excess fluid and waste material from your blood. Initially, blood enters your kidneys through the renal arteries, which are branches of the aorta — the main artery carrying oxygenated blood from your heart to the rest of your body. From there, blood moves through structures in your kidneys known as nephrons.

Each kidney contains approximately 1 million nephrons, each consisting of a tuft of capillary blood vessels (glomerulus) and tiny tubules that lead into larger collecting tubes. Each tuft of capillaries filters fluid from your bloodstream.

The filtered material, which contains both waste products and substances vital for your health, passes into the tubules. From there, waste products — urea, uric acid and creatinine — are excreted in your urine, while substances your body needs — sugar, amino acids, calcium and salts — are reabsorbed back into your bloodstream.

## New Words

amino [əˈmiːnəʊ] adj. 氨基的

aorta [eɪˈɔːtə] n. 大动脉

capillary [kəˈpɪlərɪ] n. 毛细管
　　　　　　　　adj. 毛状的，毛细作用的

creatinine [kriˈætɪniːn] n. 肌酸酐

drowsy [ˈdraʊzɪ] adj. 昏昏欲睡的，催眠的
　　　　　　　　n. 睡意

eliminate [ɪˈlɪmɪneɪt] v. 排除，消除

envelop [ɪnˈveləp] v. 包封，遮盖，包围
　　　　　　　　n. 包裹，封，包围，信封

filter [ˈfɪltər] v. 过滤，滤除，滤清

glomerulus [ɡlɒˈmerjʊləs] n. （肾）小球

inflammation [ˌɪnfləˈmeɪʃən] n. 炎症，发炎

nephron [ˈnefrɒn] n. 肾单位，肾元

overwhelming [ˌəʊvəˈhwelmɪŋ] adj. 压倒性的，无法抵抗的

oxygenate [ɒkˈsɪdʒəneɪt] v. 以氧处理，氧化

pericarditis [ˌperɪkɑːˈdaɪtɪs] n. 心包炎

retention [rɪˈtenʃən] n. 潴留

reversible [rɪˈvɜːsəbl] adj. 可逆的

spine [spaɪn] n. 脊骨，地面隆起地带

tubule [ˈtjuːbjuːl] n. 小管，细管

tuft [tʌft] n. 一丛，丛生植物，一簇
　　　　　　v. 丛生

urea [jʊˈriːə] n. 尿素

uric [ˈjʊərɪk] adj. 尿的，取自尿中的

## Exercises

**Task 8　Match the words or phrases with similar meaning in the two columns.**

A                                          B

1. peptic ulcers                    a. capillary blood vessel as nephrons in the kidney

2. *Helicobacter pylori*            b. ward the road of something through

*Note*

3. perforation     c. flow in blood vessel

4. hemorrhage     d. exceed range of natural blood pressure

5. obstruction     e. a urease-enzyme-producing bacterium

6. glomerulus     f. holes in the lining of the stomach and duodenum

7. high blood pressure     g. break a blood vessel

8. bloodstream     h. penetrate the stomach or duodenal wall

**Task 9  Choose the right answer to fill in the blanks in the passage.**

End-stage renal disease is the name for kidney failure so advanced that it cannot be reversed. The name is appropriate：the kidneys in end-stage renal disease function so poorly that they can no longer keep you ___1___ .

End-stage renal disease cannot be treated with conventional(常规的) medical treatments such as drugs. Only two treatments allow you to continue ___2___ when your kidneys stop functioning：dialysis (透析) and kidney transplantation. Dialysis is the term for several different methods of artificially filtering the blood. Kidney transplantation means replacement of the failed kidney with a working kidney from another person, called a ___3___ . Kidney transplantation is not a complete ___4___ , although many people who receive a kidney transplant are able to live much as they did before their kidneys failed. People who receive a transplant must take medication, and for the ___5___ of their lives, be monitored by a physician who specializes in kidney diseases.

The most critical part of kidney transplantation is preventing rejection of the ___6___ kidney. Different transplant centers use different drug combinations to fight rejection of a transplanted kidney. The drugs generally work by ___7___ the immune system, which is programmed to reject anything " ___8___ ", such as a new organ. You must keep follow-up appointments with your transplant team to monitor for signs of rejection. You will have regular blood and urine tests to ___9___ any signs of organ failure. One or more ultrasounds of the new kidney may be done to see if there are structural abnormalities(异常) ___10___ rejection.

1. A. live     B. living     C. life     D. alive

2. A. live     B. living     C. life     D. alive

3. A. donor     B. donate     C. recipient     D. receiver

4. A. treat     B. treatment     C. cure     D. therapy

5. A. last     B. rest     C. end     D. final

6. A. removed     B. operated     C. replaced     D. graft

7. A. compressing     B. depressing     C. suppressing     D. impressing

8. A. special     B. different     C. unique     D. foreign

9. A. search     B. seek     C. detect     D. find

10. A. suggest     B. being suggested     C. suggesting     D. suggested

## Part 4   Write and Learn

**A Recommendation Letter**

**Direction：Read the following writing sample carefully. Design and finish an imitated writing task with similar style.**

Study the following format and sample of a recommendation letter and learn how to write one.

| Format | |
|---|---|
| | Date of the letter |
| Salutation of the letter | |
| | Body of the letter |
| | Complementary close of the letter |
| | Signature |

【Sample】

June 1st, 2008

Dear Mr. Lee,

    This is to introduce Ms. May Jones, head nurse from the department of gynecology and obstetrics of our hospital who will be on business in London from April 5<sup>th</sup> to April 8<sup>th</sup>. We shall appreciate any help you can give Ms. May Jones and will always be happy to reciprocate.

Yours faithfully,

Tengfei Hospital

【Assignment】

**Write a recommendation letter according to the following information.**

兹介绍我院儿科护士长许华女士前往纽约市的希尔顿医院出差三周,请接洽。

秋阳医科大学

2008 年 5 月 5 日

# Part 5  Prefixes, Suffixes & Roots

**Urinary System (泌尿系统)**

| 汉语(英语) | 常 用 词 根 | 例　词 |
|---|---|---|
| 尿(urine) | urin(o)-;<br>ur(o)- | urinary 尿的;urinogenital 泌尿生殖的;<br>hematuria 血尿;polyuria 多尿症 |
| 肾(kidney) | ren(o)-;<br>nephr(o)- | nephritis 肾炎;suprarenal 肾上的;<br>renovascular 肾血管的;hydronephrosis 肾盂积水 |
| 膀胱(bladder) | vesic(o)-; cyst(o)- | vesical 膀胱的;rectovesical 直肠膀胱的;<br>cystitis 膀胱炎;cystostomy 膀胱造瘘术 |
| 尿道(urethra) | urethr(o)-; meat(o)- | urethritis 尿道炎; urethroscopy 尿道镜检查;<br>meatotomy 尿道口切开术;meatorrhaphy 尿道口缝合术 |
| 睾丸(testis) | test(o)-;<br>testicul(o)-;<br>orchi(o)-;<br>didym(o)- | testosterone 睾酮;testicular 睾丸的;<br>orchitis 睾丸炎;epididymis 附睾 |
| 前列腺<br>(prostate) | prostat(o)- | prostatic 前列腺的;prostatitis 前列腺炎;<br>prostatectomy 前列腺切除术;prostatalgia 前列腺痛 |

*Note*

续表

| 汉语（英语） | 常用词根 | 例　　词 |
|---|---|---|
| 肾盂<br>（renal pelvis） | pelvi(o)-；pyel(o)- | pyelonephritis 肾盂肾炎；<br>pyelography 肾盂造影术 |

**Task 10　Learn the prefixes, suffixes or roots in the table by heart and then choose the best answer to finish the exercises.**

1. Fill in the blank with the combining part for the medical term "尿道造影术": _____ -graphy.

A. urino　　　　　B. ureter　　　　　C. urethro　　　　　D. urethra

2. The correct spelling form for the word "尿道炎" is _____.

A. uteritis　　　　B. urinitis　　　　C. ureteritis　　　　D. urethritis

3. The correct spelling form for the word "肾盂积水" is _____.

A. hydrorenosis　B. hydronephrosis　C. hydrorenitis　　D. hydronephritis

4. The word with Chinese meaning as "血尿" is _____.

A. hematuria　　　B. hemaurine　　　C. hemaurinati　　　D. hemaurinary

5. Inflammation of the prostate is given the term as _____.

A. orchitis　　　　B. orchotitis　　　C. prostatitis　　　D. prostatotitis

6. Which word in the following has the meaning of "no urine"? _____

A. anuria　　　　　B. polyuria　　　　C. anurine　　　　　D. polyurine

7. Inflammation of the testis is given the term as _____.

A. epididymoorchitis　B. orchitis　　C. epididymitis　　D. epididymis

8. Fill in the blank with the combining part for the medical term "膀胱造影术": _____ -graphy.

A. gall bladder　　B. bladder　　　　C. vesico　　　　　D. cysto

9. Which word in the following has nothing to do with "睾丸"? _____

A. testiculo-　　　B. testo-　　　　　C. cysto-　　　　　D. orchi-

10. The correct spelling form for the word "膀胱输尿管的" is _____.

A. cystocoureteral　B. vesicoureteral　C. vesicourethral　D. bladderureteral

# Unit 8　The Musculoskeletal System

## Learning Objectives:

To remember some key English words related to the musculoskeletal system.

To understand the conversation about enema and talk about the topic.

To read and understand the main ideas and the details of the passages about the musculoskeletal system.

To learn to write an application letter with the help of the given sample writing.

To learn by heart some word roots, prefixes and suffixes about the musculoskeletal system.

## Part 1　Look and Learn

**Warming-up 1: Look at the following picture, talk about them and then finish Task 1.**

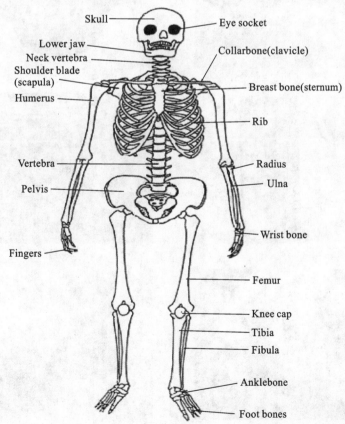

## New Words

vertebra ['vɜːtɪbrə] n. 椎骨

collarbone ['kɒləbəʊn] n. 锁骨

humerus ['hjuːmərəs] n. 肱骨

radius ['reɪdɪəs] n. 桡骨

ulna ['ʌlnə] n. 尺骨

femur ['fiːmə(r)] n. 股骨

tibia ['tɪbɪə] n. 胫骨

fibula ['fɪbjʊlə] n. 腓骨

**Task 1　Match the words in the left column with the explanations in the right column.**

| 1. humerus | A. the outer and slightly shorter of the two bones of the human forearm |
| --- | --- |
| 2. radius | B. the bone that extends from the shoulder to the elbow |
| 3. ulna | C. the inner and longer of the two bones of the human forearm |
| 4. tibia | D. the outer bone of the two bones in the lower part of your leg |
| 5. fibula | E. the inner bone of the two bones in the lower part of your leg |

**Warming-up 2：Look at the following pictures about medical instruments，talk about them and then finish Task 2.**

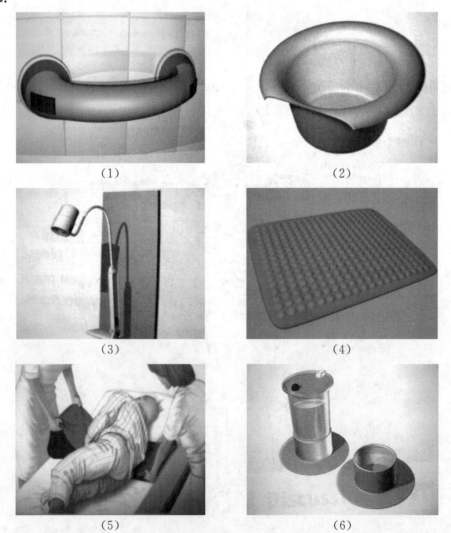

(1)

(2)

(3)

(4)

(5)

(6)

## New Words

slide [slaɪd] v. 滑动

vomit ['vɒmɪt] v. 呕吐

mat [mæt] n. 席子，垫子

non-tip adj. 固定的

**Task 2　Match the picture number with the proper English and Chinese meaning.**

| Picture number | English | Chinese |
|---|---|---|
| | slide sheet | 移动床单 |
| | vomit bowl | 痰盂 |
| | light | 灯 |
| | grab bar | 扶手、抓条 |
| | non-slip mat | 防滑垫 |
| | non-tip cup | 不倒杯 |

# Part 2　Listen and Learn

## Situation Dialogue：Enema

**Task 3　Listen to the audio episode one and fill in the missing words referring to the original text. Then check your writing against the original.**

Nurse：Hi，Mr. John. How are you today?

Patient：Not bad. How are you?

Nurse：Good. I hear you've been constipated for a few days.

Patient：Yes. I haven't had bowel movement at least 4 days so my abdomen feels distended and painful. I 1._____ but it doesn't work.

Nurse：That must be uncomfortable. Dr. Peter 2._____ an enema for you.

Patient：Oh，what is 3._____? Will it hurt?

Nurse：An enema is a tube of liquid inserted into the rectum through the anus to help your bowel movements. It won't hurt. I am sure you can 4._____ it.

Patient：OK，I hope so. What should I do now?

Nurse：You should go to the bathroom first. I'll go to prepare the stuff and come back later.

扫码听
对话 1

**Task 4　Listen to the audio episode two and complete the answers according to the questions.**

1. What does the nurse ask the patient show to her?

The nurse asks the patient to show her _____ bracelet.

2. How should the patient lie?

The patient should take off his pants to the knees and lie _____.

3. How long is the patient asked to keep the position?

The nurse asks the patient to keep the position for _____ minutes.

扫码听
对话 2

Note

## Part 3   Read and Learn

扫码听
课文 A

Passage A

### Rise in Broken Bones in Children

Across the country, doctors are reporting a steady increase in the number of children with broken bones.

"The fact of the matter is that children are breaking bones all over," said Dr. Laura Tosi, a pediatric orthopedic surgeon in Washington, D. C. "It's a very high incidence of elbow fractures, as well as fractures in the mid-part of the arm, and in the hand." A recently published study by the Mayo Clinic found that over the last 30 years the number of forearm fractures in that city has climbed more than 32 percent in boys, and 56 percent in girls. Researchers say they are not sure why the fracture rate is rising. But they suspect a major reason is that children are not getting enough calcium, which is essential for strong bones.

"Calcium deficiency is the major dietary deficiency in America's children today," says Dr. Duane Alexander. According to statistics from the U. S. Department of Agriculture, 86 percent of teenage girls and 64 percent of teenage boys are "calcium deficient"; in other words, they lack the recommended daily amount (RDA) of calcium, which is 1,300 milligrams, the equivalent of about four 8-ounce glasses of milk a day.

"Over the last 20 to 30 years, there's been a shift away from milk as the standard drink at meals and for increased use of soft drinks and juices, and other drinks by kids at all ages," said Alexander. "Without adequate milk consumption, it's virtually impossible for a child to get the calcium intake they need in their diets," said Alexander. And a child has critical calcium needs.

Calcium is effective at building bones, but researchers say only until the age of 20. After that, regardless of how much you take, bone mass does not increase, and the slow process of bone loss soon begins. The best calcium can do for adults is to slow the loss of bone. So calcium-deficient children today are at much greater risk of developing osteoporosis as they age, and even more broken bones.

## New Words

pediatric [ˌpiːdɪˈætrɪk] adj. 小儿科的

orthopedic [ˌɔːθəˈpiːdɪk] adj. 整形外科的

surgeon [ˈsɜːdʒən] n. 外科医生

incidence [ˈɪnsɪdəns] n. 发生率

fracture [ˈfræktʃə(r)] n. 断裂,骨折
　　　　　　　　　　　　v. 破裂,使破裂

calcium [ˈkælsɪəm] n. 钙

essential [ɪˈsenʃl] adj. 基本的,必要的
　　　　　　　　n. 本质,要素

deficiency [dɪˈfɪʃənsɪ] n. 缺陷,缺乏

dietary [ˈdaɪətərɪ] adj. 饮食的,饭食的
　　　　　　　n. 规定的食物,食谱

equivalent [ɪˈkwɪvələnt] adj. (价值、数量等方面)相等的

Note

n. 对等的人(或事)

adequate ['ædɪkwət] adj. 充足的,适当的

consumption [kən'sʌmpʃn] n. 消费,消耗

virtually ['vɜːtʃʊəlɪ] adv. 几乎,事实上,实质上

critical ['krɪtɪkl] adj. 决定性的,关键性的

osteoporosis [ˌɒstiəupə'rəusɪs] n. 骨质疏松症

**Task 5    Fill in the blanks with the words given below and change the word forms if necessary.**

1. She gave me the phone number for the nearest pharmacy so I could make arrangements with our _____(pediatric) to call in prescriptions.

2. So go back to my description of _____(orthopedic), I would be fixing a kid's hip.

3. He is reputed to be the best heart _____(surgical) in the country.

4. You've _____(fracture) a rib, maybe more than one.

5. Of course in the reversible case, you're always pushing against an external pressure, which is _____(essential) equal to the internal pressure.

6. Deaf people are sometimes treated as being mentally _____(deficiency).

7. They felt slighted by not being _____(adequately) consulted.

8. The three bombs were _____(virtual) identical.

9. She kept vigil at the bedside of her _____(critical) ill son.

10. Perhaps soy can help prevent _____(osteoporotic), mumps or even chicken pox.

**Task 6    Choose the correct answer according to the passage.**

1. What is the passage mainly about? _____

A. the treatment of broken bones

B. a hot topic in pediatrics

C. osteoporosis can be cured if we drink more milk

D. the reason of rising in broken bones in children

2. How much RDA of calcium that children lack? _____

A. 1,300 mg        B. 1,200 mg        C. 1,400 mg        D. 1,100 mg

3. Which of the followings is the way of avoiding calcium deficiency? _____

A. doing less physical exercises

B. drinking more soft drink

C. drinking adequate milk

D. avoiding the swelling of the joint

4. Researchers suspect the major reason that the fracture rate is rising is that _____.

A. children are more likely to develop osteoporosis

B. children cannot pay for enough the calcium supplements

C. children are not getting enough calcium

D. children grow and develop faster

5. Which of the following statements can we infer from the passage? _____

A. We can take calcium supplements after the age of 20 to increase bone mass

B. Children can drink adequate milk for lowering the risk of developing osteoporosis

C. Calcium deficiency is the major dietary deficiency in children

D. Adults are less likely to have osteoporosis

*Note*

**Task 7  Arrange the following steps in proper sequence based on the medical procedure.**

_____ Spinal immobilization is the highest priority; do not move casualty unless in danger.

_____ Support casualty's head and neck at all times. Place hands on side of the head until other support arranged.

_____ Check breathing and pulse.

_____ Apply a cervical or improvised collar to minimize neck movement.

_____ Wait for an ambulance.

_____ Give reassurance: calm casualty.

## New Words

spinal ['spaɪnl] adj. 脊柱的，与脊柱有关的

immobilization [ɪˌməʊbɪlaɪ'zeɪʃən] n. 固定

priority [praɪ'ɒrətɪ] n. 优先，优先权；(时间，序上的)先，前

cervical ['sɜːvɪkl] adj. 颈的

improvise ['ɪmprəvaɪz] v. 临时提供，临时凑成

minimize ['mɪnɪmaɪz] v. 把……减至最少

扫码听 课文 B

**Passage B**

**Bone Fracture**

When external forces are applied to bone, it has the potential to fail. Fractures occur when bone cannot withstand those external forces. When fracture happens, the integrity of the bone has been lost and the bone structure fails.

There are many classifications of fractures according to characteristics such as where they occur and their appearance. A closed fracture means the skin around the fractured bone is not broken. An open one includes a break in the skin, revealing the bone and making the wound more susceptible to infection. A fracture is called complete if the break is the whole way through the bone, and incomplete (or greenstick) if the break is partial. Greenstick fractures are more commonly seen in children. Stress fractures are small cracks in a bone that occur over time as a result of repeated activities that put stress on the bone. According to the way the fracture line goes across the bone, we have transverse fracture, oblique fracture or spiral fracture. If the fracture is in multiple pieces, it is comminuted fracture. Actually, a person can have just one fracture or multiple fractures at the same time.

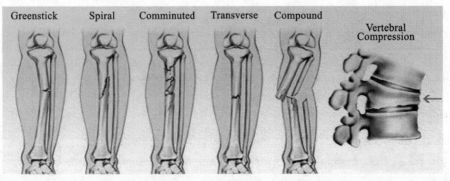

Generally speaking, a bone fracture results in pain, swelling, and sometimes, bruising from internal bleeding. The patient cannot bear weight or pressure on the injured area, and may be unable

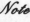

to move it with severe pain. The soft tissues around the broken bone may also be injured. The area around or below the fracture may feel numb or paralyzed due to a loss of pulse in that area.

A bone fracture is diagnosed by a physical examination and X-rays of the injured area. However, some types of fractures are difficult to see on an X-ray. In this case, your doctor may order other diagnostic imaging tests, such as computed tomography, magnetic resonance imaging, or bone scans. Open fractures require additional laboratory tests to determine whether blood has been lost and if there is infection.

Initial treatment for fractures of the arms, legs, hands and feet in the field include splinting the extremity in the position it is found, elevation and ice. Immobilization will be very helpful with initial pain control. For injuries of the neck and back, first responders or paramedics may choose to place the injured person on a long board and in a neck collar to protect the spinal cord from potential injury.

Surgery on fractures is very much dependent on what bone is broken and where it is broken. The bones are manipulated by surgeons so that alignment is restored and a cast is placed to hold the bones in that alignment. Sometimes, the bones are broken in such a way that they need to have metal hardware inserted to hold them in place. Depending on the fracture, some of these pieces of metal are permanent, and some are temporary until the healing of the bone is complete and surgically removed at a later time.

## New Words

alignment [ə'laɪnmənt] n. 排成直线，队列
bruise [bruːz] n. 淤伤，擦伤
　　　　　　v. 打伤，撞伤
comminute ['kɒmɪnjuːt] v. 使成粉末，粉碎，分割
immobilization [ɪˌməʊbɪlaɪ'zeɪʃən] n. 固定
magnetic [mæg'netɪk] adj. 磁的，有磁性的
manipulate [mə'nɪpjʊleɪt] vt. (熟练地)操作，使用
multiple ['mʌltɪpl] adj. 多样的，多重的
oblique [ə'bliːk] adj. 倾斜的
paralyze ['pærəlaɪz] v. 使瘫痪，使麻痹
paramedic [ˌpærə'medɪk] n. 护理人员
resonance ['rezənəns] n. 共鸣，回声，共振
surgery ['sɜːdʒərɪ] n. 外科，外科学，手术室，诊疗室
spiral ['spaɪərəl] adj. 螺旋形的
　　　　　　n. 螺旋
　　　　　　v. 盘旋
splint [splɪnt] n. 薄金属片，夹板
　　　　　v. 用夹板夹
tomography [təʊ'mɒɡrəfɪ] n. X线断层摄影术
transverse ['trænz'vɜːs] adj. 横向的，横断的

*Note*

## Exercises

**Task 8  Match the words or phrases with similar meaning in the two columns.**

| A | B |
|---|---|
| 1. initial | a. everlasting |
| 2. poisonous | b. nursing staff |
| 3. pulmonary | c. operation |
| 4. fracture | d. man-made |
| 5. immobilization | e. first, beginning |
| 6. permanent | f. toxic |
| 7. paramedic | g. related or about lung(s) |
| 8. surgery | h. continuous |
| 9. artificial | i. break |
| 10. sequential | j. fixation |

**Task 9  Choose the right answer to fill in the blanks in the passage.**

Water is absolutely vital to good health. Next to air, water is the most essential(基本的) element to our survival(生存).  __1__  it, humans would die in a few days.

Water makes up(组成) two-thirds of our bodies; 95% of human brain is made up of water; while blood is 82% and lungs is 90%. It is obvious that water plays an important  __2__  in maintaining (维持) our health. It is  __3__  that drinking 5 glasses of water daily decreases the risk of breast cancer  __4__  79%. However, most people drink  __5__  than the eight recommended glasses each day. Almost one-third of people drink  __6__  water at all.

Why is drinking enough water  __7__  important? A minor water shortage can  __8__  to headaches and sleepiness, while long-lasting shortage of water can cause high blood pressure and  __9__  serious problems.

Drinking water helps our bodies in a  __10__  of ways. It helps us get rid of wastes, carry nutrients, and regulate body temperature. Also, water gives our skin a healthy smooth.

1. A. Despite          B. Except          C. Without
2. A. rule             B. role            C. duty
3. A. reporting        B. reported        C. being reported
4. A. to               B. by              C. for
5. A. fewer            B. more            C. much
6. A. no               B. little          C. less
7. A. such             B. so              C. as
8. A. cause            B. lead            C. make
9. A. other            B. the other       C. another
10. A. variable        B. various         C. variety

## Part 4   Write and Learn

### An Application Letter

**Direction：Read the following writing sample carefully. Design and finish an imitated writing task with similar style.**

求职信是十分实用的一种应用文。第一段：直奔主题说明写信目的，即求职，以及所求职位。第二段：中心段，说明求职条件，即所学专业、最后学历，以及工作经历，包括兼职或做过的工作。第三段：结尾段，要求面试，盼望回信，写清楚联系方式，并表示感谢。

【Sample】

假定你是李明，某报社招聘新闻信件的编辑，你写信求职。

1. 你毕业于四川大学新闻专业，硕士学位。

2. 你曾担任校报体育编辑；现为华西出版社写稿，并担任编辑。

Dear personnel manager，

I notice your ad for a newsletter editor in the October 29<sup>th</sup> *China Daily*. Because writing and publication work have long been interests of mine，I wish to apply for this position.

I believe that both my education and work experience qualify me for the job. In 2011，I graduated from Sichuan University；at the same time，I earned my master degree with a major in journalism and a minor in English. While in school，I was the sports editor on the campus newspaper. Since graduation，I have written and edited the monthly bulletin of the Huaxi Press.

I am currently available for an interview any weekday after 3：00 pm. You can reach me at my home phone，855-7382，and any day after 3：00 pm. I'm looking forward to hearing from you and appreciate your consideration of my application.

Sincerely yours，<br>Li Ming

【Assignment】

假定你是王璐，某医学院护理专业大四学生，即将毕业，某医院正在招聘护士，请写一封求职信。

## Part 5   Prefixes, Suffixes & Roots

**Diseases(1)**

| 汉语（英语） | 常用词根 | 例　　　词 |
| --- | --- | --- |
| 异常（abnormal） | dys- | dysplasia 发育异常；dyspepsia 消化不良；dyspnea 呼吸困难；dysuria 排尿困难；dysfunction 功能失调 |
| 不良（bad） | mal- | maladaptive 不适应的；malformation 畸形；malfunction 功能障碍；malnutrition 营养不良 |
| 慢（slow） | brady- | bradypnea 呼吸过慢；bradycardia 心动过缓 |
| 快（rapid） | tachy- | tachycardia 心动过速；tachypnea 呼吸急促；tachymeter 速度计（速测仪）；tachyuria 排尿急促 |

| 汉语(英语) | 常用词根 | 例 词 |
| --- | --- | --- |
| 扩张(dilation) | -cele | omphalocele 脐突出；hydrocele 积水(阴囊积水)；bronchocele 支气管囊肿；hematocele 血肿 |
| 发炎(inflammation) | -itis | cholecystitis 胆囊炎；nephritis 肾炎；neuritis 神经炎；myocarditis 心肌炎；phlebitis 静脉炎 |
| 出血(bleeding) | -rrhagia -staxis | colonorrhagia 结肠出血；cystorrhagia 膀胱出血；enterostaxis 肠渗血；bronchostaxis 支气管出血 |
| 溢出(discharge) | -rrhea | diarrhea 腹泻(痢疾)；glycorrhea 糖溢；gastrorrhea 胃液溢出；hemorrhea 大出血 |
| 溶解(dissolving) | -lysis | hydrolysis 水解；hemolysis 溶血(血细胞溶解)；proteolytic 蛋白水解的；bacteriolysis 溶菌作用 |
| 嗜好(like) | -philia | hydrophilia 亲水性；pharmacophilia 嗜药性 |
| 恐惧(fear) | -phobia | hydrophobia 恐水病；aerophobia 高空恐惧症；carcinomatophobia 癌症恐惧症 |
| 下垂(dropping) | -ptosis | gastroptosis 胃下垂；nephroptosis 肾下垂；gastroenteroptosis 胃肠下垂；cardioptosis 心脏下垂 |
| 病毒(virus) | viro- | virocytology 病毒细胞学；virogene 病毒基因；viromembrane 病毒膜；virostatic 病毒抑制药 |

**Task 10  Learn the prefixes, suffixes or roots in the table by heart and then choose the best answer to finish the exercises.**

1. The Chinese meaning for "dysuria" is _____.

A. 排尿困难　　　B. 发育异常　　　C. 消化不良　　　D. 呼吸困难

2. Fill in the blank with the combining part for the medical term "心动过缓"：_____ - cardia.

A. tachy　　　B. brady　　　C. dys　　　D. mal

3. The Chinese meaning for "tachypnea" is _____.

A. 心动过速　　　B. 心动过缓　　　C. 呼吸急促　　　D. 呼吸过慢

4. The English term for "结肠出血" is _____.

A. bronchostaxis　　B. enterostaxis　　C. cystorrhagia　　D. colonorrhagia

5. The English term for "支气管囊肿" is _____.

A. omphalocele　　B. hydrocele　　C. hematocele　　D. bronchocele

6. The word which has something to do with "dropping" is _____.

A. hepatitis　　　B. gastritis　　　C. gastroptosis　　　D. nephritis

7. To choose a word for "心肌炎", its correct spelling is _____.

A. bronchitis　　B. myocarditis　　C. phlebitis　　D. cholecystitis

8. The following words have the meaning of virus except _____.

A. bacteriolysis　　B. virocytology　　C. viromembrane　　D. virogene

9. Which word has the meaning of "胃肠下垂"? _____

A. gastroenteroptosis B. gastroptosis　　C. nephroptosis　　D. cardioptosis

10. The following words have the meaning of speeding except _____.

A. tachycardia　　B. bradypnea　　C. tachypnea　　D. tachyuria

# Unit 9 The Oral Cavity

## Learning Objectives:

To remember some key English words related to the oral cavity.

To understand the conversation about health education and talk about the topic.

To read and understand the main ideas and the details of the passages about the oral cavity.

To learn to write an essay about blood donation with the help of the given sample writing.

To learn by heart some word roots, prefixes and suffixes about disease.

## Part 1 Look and Learn

**Warming -up 1: Look at the following picture, talk about them and then finish Task 1.**

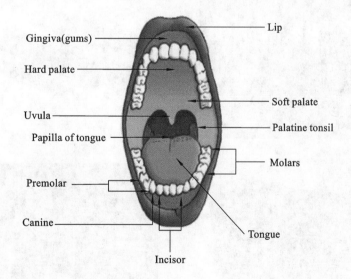

## New Words

gingiva [dʒɪnˈdʒaɪvə] n. 齿龈

uvula [ˈjuːvjʊlə] n. 悬雍垂

papilla [pəˈpɪlə] n. 小乳头状突起

palatine [ˈpælətaɪn] adj. 上颚的

premolar [ˈpriːˈməʊlə(r)] n. 前臼齿

molar [ˈməʊlə(r)] n. 臼齿

*Note*

canine ['keɪnaɪn] n. 犬齿

incisor [ɪn'saɪzə(r)] n. 门齿

**Task 1** **Match the words in the left column with the explanations in the right column.**

| | |
|---|---|
| 1. tonsil | A. the soft part in the mouth that moves around, used for tasting, swallowing, speaking, etc. |
| 2. lip | B. either of two masses of lymphatic tissue one on each side of the oral pharynx |
| 3. tongue | C. the top part of the inside of the mouth |
| 4. palate | D. either of the two soft edges at the opening to the mouth |
| 5. canine | E. one of the four pointed conical teeth (two in each jaw) located between the incisors and the premolars |

**Warming-up 2: Look at the following pictures about medical instruments, talk about them and then finish Task 2.**

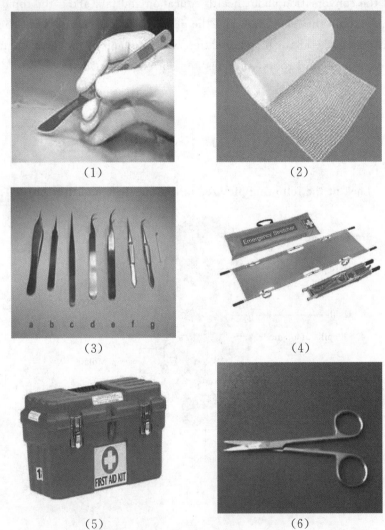

(1)　　　　　　　　　　　(2)

(3)　　　　　　　　　　　(4)

(5)　　　　　　　　　　　(6)

## New Words

scissors ['sɪzəz] n. 剪刀

scalpel ['skælpəl] n. 外科手术刀

forceps ['fɔːseps] n. 医用镊子

cke
**Task 2  Match the picture number with the proper English and Chinese meaning.**

| Picture number | English | Chinese |
| --- | --- | --- |
| | stretcher | 担架 |
| | first-aid kit | 急救箱 |
| | scissors | 剪刀 |
| | bandage | 绷带 |
| | scalpel | 外科手术刀 |
| | forceps | 医用镊子 |

# Part 2  Listen and Learn

## Situation Dialogue：Health Education

**Task 3  Listen to the audio episode one and fill in the missing words referring to the original text. Then check your writing against the original.**

Nurse：Hi，Mrs. Jenny. How are you today?

Patient：Good. How are you?

Nurse：Very good. Thank you. I'd like to talk about your 1. _____ management before your discharge.

Patient：Oh，thanks. I am really worrying about the complication of the diabetes after I go back home.

Nurse：I understand it's not easy for you to manage it now，so we need to 2. _____ you first.

Patient：I think so.

Nurse：OK，let's start. There are two types of diabetes，type 1 and type 2. Do you know what type you have?

Patient：Type 2. It's also called the non-insulin-dependent diabetes. And the doctor suggested that I take the 3. _____ injections.

Nurse：Good. Can you tell me how many units have been 4. _____ for you?

Patient：Four units of 5. _____ insulin. But I am not sure.

**Task 4  Listen to the audio episode two and complete the answers according to the questions.**

1. When should the patient inject the insulin?

   Remember to inject the insulin 30 minutes _____.

2. Why do most diabetics use insulin pen?

   Most diabetics use insulin pen because its prefilled devices are _____ for them.

3. According to doctors' orders，what must the patient do in case of hyperglycemia?

   The patient must control her _____ according to doctors' orders in case of hyperglycemia.

扫码听 对话1

扫码听 对话2

*Note*

# Part 3　Read and Learn

**Passage A**

### Gingivitis and Periodontal Disease

The first section of the mouth is known as the oral cavity. This space is bordered in the front and to the sides by two arches, which contain the teeth. The oral cavity also contains the tongue, hard and soft palates, uvula, and gums. This entire structure is also called the mouth; the structures within the mouth allow us to taste and chew food, to swallow food and drink, and to manipulate the air that comes up from the voice box so that we can form words.

Some common problems related to the oral cavity include bad breath, tooth decay, gum disease, oral cancer, and mouth sores. To prevent these problems, people can brush their teeth twice a day and floss daily, get oral cancer screenings at least once a year, avoid smoking, eat healthy foods, and change their toothbrush about every two months.

Gingivitis, or inflammation of the gums, usually comes before periodontitis, or gum disease. In the early stage of gingivitis, bacteria in plaque build up, causing the gums to become inflamed and to easily bleed during tooth brushing. Although the gums may be irritated, the teeth are still firmly planted in their sockets. No irreversible bone or other tissue damage has occurred at this stage.

When gingivitis is untreated, it can lead to periodontitis. In a person with periodontitis, the inner layer of the gum and bone pull away from the teeth and form pockets. These small spaces between teeth and gums collect debris and can become infected. The body's immune system fights the bacteria as the plaque spreads and grows below the gum line.

Toxins or poisons produced by the bacteria in plaque as well as the body's "good" enzymes involved in fighting infections — start to break down the bone and connective tissue that hold teeth in place. As the disease progresses, the pockets deepen and more gum tissues and bones are destroyed. When this happens, teeth are no longer anchored in place, they become loose, and tooth loss occurs. The gums appear to be pale in color, instead of a healthy pink. Gum disease is the leading cause of tooth loss in adults.

People can prevent gingivitis and periodontitis by brushing their teeth every day, flossing, and abstaining from bad oral habits, such as smoking.

## New Words

cavity [ˈkævətɪ] n. 腔

arch [ɑːtʃ] n. 弓，弓形

swallow [ˈswɒləʊ] v. 吞，咽

manipulate [məˈnɪpjʊleɪt] v. 操作

gingivitis [ˌdʒɪndʒɪˈvaɪtɪs] n. 牙龈炎

inflame [ɪnˈfleɪm] v. 发炎

irritate [ˈɪrɪteɪt] v. 使疼痛，使发炎

decay [dɪˈkeɪ] n. 衰败

pocket [ˈpɒkɪt] n. 小区域

abstain [əbˈsteɪn] v. 戒除

*Note*

**Task 5   Fill in the blanks with the words given below and change the word forms if necessary.**

1. Computers are very efficient at _____(manipulate) information.

2. The doctor has advised him to _____(abstain) from smoking.

3. The vegetables have begun to _____(decay).

4. Drinking milk regularly can improve physical quality and enhance ability to _____ (immune).

5. Some drugs can _____(irritate) the lining of the stomach.

6. Always chew food well before _____(swallow) it.

7. Men over 55 years old should be regularly _____(screen) for prostate cancer.

8. After the operation you may find it difficult to _____(chew) and swallow.

9. When you have measles, you must stay at home or you will _____(infect) the class.

10. His comments have _____(inflame) teachers all over the country.

**Task 6   Choose the correct answer according to the passage.**

1. What do oral cavity contain? _____

A. teeth, uvula

B. tongue, gums

C. hard and soft palates

D. A, B, and C

2. What's the common problems related to the oral cavity? _____

A. tooth decay

B. gum disease

C. A, B, and D

D. mouth sores

3. How to prevent oral problems? _____

A. never brush teeth

B. get oral cancer screenings regularly

C. keep smoking

D. seldom change toothbrush

4. When would periodontitis or gum disease come? _____

A. When gingivitis is untreated, it can lead to periodontitis

B. Periodontitis or gum disease often comes before gingivitis

C. If people brush and floss their teeth every day, they would get gum disease

D. When people abstain from bad oral habits such as smoking, they can get periodontitis

5. How to prevent gingivitis and periodontitis? _____

A. never brush your teeth

B. keep smoking

C. eat imbalanced meals

D. visit your dentist regularly for professional cleanings

**Task 7   Arrange the following steps about upper limb injury in proper sequence based on the medical procedure.**

_____ If possible gently bend the casualty's arm at the elbow so that her forearm is across her

*Note*

95

chest and place soft padding between the fracture site and her body.

_____ Take the casualty to hospital.

_____ For additional support, secure the casualty's arm to her trunk by applying a broad-fold bandage right around her arm and trunk. Avoid the fracture site.

_____ Support her arm with an arm sling.

扫码听
课文 B

### Passage B

#### Young Hit by Mouth Cancer Increase

Increasing numbers of young people are being hit by mouth cancer, sparking new warnings about the disease.

Mouth cancer was once considered to mostly affect older men, but it is now becoming more common in younger people and women.

It is possible that binge-drinking and smoking could be helping to fuel rising rates of the disease as these are key risk factors.

Now the British Dental Health Foundation (BDHF) is warning people of all ages that they need to start checking their mouths regularly if rising rates of mouth cancer are to be stopped.

The ratio of women to men suffering mouth cancer has grown by a third in the last 10 years, although men are still twice as likely to develop the disease.

Mouth cancer is sometimes called oral cancer and can affect the lips, tongue, cheeks and throat.

Every year in the UK, there are 4,300 new cases diagnosed and 1,700 deaths.

The most common causes of mouth cancer are smoking and drinking alcohol to excess — people who do both are up to 30 times more likely to develop the condition than those who do not.

Having a poor diet is also linked to the disease.

But the BDHF said about 25% of mouth cancer cases in younger people involved none of these common risk factors. The foundation said this meant that it was vital people learnt to be aware of the possible symptoms, even if they led a healthy lifestyle.

## New Words

spark [spɑːk] v. 激起

fuel [fjʊəl] v. 加剧

ratio ['reɪʃɪəʊ] n. 比率

diagnose ['daɪəgnəʊz] v. 诊断

vital ['vaɪtəl] adj. 至关重要的

binge [bɪndʒ] n. 放纵

foundation [faʊn'deɪʃən] n. 基金会

excess [ɪk'ses] n. 超额量

involve [ɪn'vɒlv] v. 涉及

aware [ə'weə(r)] adj. 意识到的

## Exercises

**Task 8  Match the words or phrases with similar meaning in the two columns.**

| A | B |
|---|---|
| 1. spark | a. indulgence |
| 2. fuel | b. organization |
| 3. ratio | c. intensify |
| 4. diagnose | d. arouse |
| 5. vital | e. proportion |
| 6. binge | f. realizing |
| 7. foundation | g. include |
| 8. excess | h. essential |
| 9. involve | i. extra |
| 10. aware | j. analyze |

**Task 9  Choose the right answer to fill in the blanks in the passage.**

It was the kind of research that gave insight into how flu strains could mutate so quickly. The same branch of research concluded in 2005 that 1918 flu started in birds before passing to humans, parsing this animal-human __1__ could provide clues to __2__ the next potential super-flu, which already has a name: H5N1, also known as avian flu or bird flu.

This potential killer also has a number: 59%. According to the WHO, nearly three-fifths of the people who __3__ H5N1 since 2003 died from the virus, which was first reported __4__ humans in Hong Kong in 1997 before a more serious __5__ occurred in Southeast Asia between 2003 and 2004. (It has since spread to Africa and Europe.) Some researchers argue that those morality numbers are exaggerated because WHO only __6__ cases in which victims are sick enough to go to hospitals for treatment. __7__, compared that with the worldwide mortality rate of 1918 pandemic, it may have killed roughly 50 million people, but that was only 10% of the number of people infected, according to a 2006 estimate.

H5N1's saving grace — and the only reason we're not running around masked up in public right now — is that the strain doesn't jump from birds to humans, or from humans to humans, easily. There have been just over 600 cases (and 359 deaths) since 2003. But __8__ its lethality, and the chance it could turn into something far more than transmissible, one might expect H5N1 research to be exploding, with labs __9__ the virus's molecular components to understand how it spreads between animals and __10__ to humans, and hoping to discover a vaccine that could head off a pandemic.

1. A. rejection       B. interface       C. complement       D. contamination
2. A. be stopped      B. stopping        C. being stopped    D. having stopped
3. A. mutated         B. effected        C. infected         D. contracted
4. A. in              B. on              C. with             D. from
5. A. trigger         B. launch          C. outbreak         D. outcome
6. A. counts          B. amounts to      C. accounts for     D. accumulates
7. A. Thereafter      B. Thereby         C. Furthermore      D. Still
8. A. given           B. regarding       C. in spite of      D. speaking of
9. A. parses          B. parsed          C. parsing          D. to parse
10. A. potently       B. absolutely      C. potentially      D. important

*Note*

## Part 4  Write and Learn

### Essay Writing（1）

**Direction：Read the following writing sample carefully. Design and finish an imitated writing task with similar style.**

从一般意义上讲,英语议论文由于所阐释的重点不一样,各自具备不同的特点和板块结构。在考试中英语议论文一直都是考试的重点,也是学生学习英语必须掌握的一种实用技能。英语议论文常见类型包括总结类议论文、解决问题类议论文、个人观点类议论文和对比类议论文。总结类议论文常为三段式:第一段,简明扼要地点明要论述的话题,并稍加阐述;第二段,中心段,主要分析原因或说明意义、实施的方法;第三段,常称为结尾段,对所阐述的内容加以总结概括。

【Sample】

Keep Health

Outline：1. 健康十分重要。

　　　　2. 怎样保持健康。

　　　　3. 总结。

As a proverb says, " No one knows the value of health until he loses it. " In other words, nothing is more valuable than health. If we are sick, it is impossible for us to pursue our career effectively.

Now that we know that health is the resource of our energy, what should we do to maintain our health? First, we should take exercise every day to strengthen our muscles, such as jogging every day, playing tennis at regular time, or climbing on holidays. Second, we should be in a good mood every day. If we get up early, we can breathe fresh air and see the sunrise. This habit can do wonders for our outlook on life. Last, there is a proverb that says, "Prevention is better than cure. " If we pay close attention to our health, we can avoid getting sick.

From what has been discussed above, we may safely come to the conclusion that health is vital for us. If we want to make our dreams come true, health is the most important ingredient of our success.

【Assignment】

Blood Donation

Outline：1. 无偿献血的人越来越多。

　　　　2. 无偿献血的意义。

　　　　3. 总结。

## Part 5  Prefixes, Suffixes & Roots

**Diseases（2）**

| 汉语（英语） | 常用词根 | 例　　词 |
| --- | --- | --- |
| 肿瘤（tumor） | onc(h)-；onc(o)- -oma | oncogene 致癌或癌基因；oncology 肿瘤学；oncocyte 肿瘤细胞；oncogen 致肿瘤物；myofibroma 肌纤维瘤；melanoma 黑色素瘤 |

续表

| 汉语(英语) | 常用词根 | 例　词 |
|---|---|---|
| 疾病(disease) | path(o)-<br>-pathy | pathogen 病原体；histopathology 组织病理学；<br>pathoanatomy 病理解剖学；gastropathy 胃病<br>neuropathy 神经病；nephropathy 肾病 |
| 脓(pus) | py(o)- | pyocyst 脓囊肿；pyorrhea 脓漏(脓溢)；<br>pyogenesis 化脓；pyuria 脓尿 |
| 发烧(fever) | pyr(o)-<br>pyret(o)- | pyretic 发热的；pyrexia 发热；<br>pyretology 热病学；hyperpyrexia 高热；<br>pyrogenous 高热所产生的；pyretolysis 退烧 |
| 硬化(hardening) | scler(o)- | sclerosis 硬化症；arteriosclerosis 动脉硬化症；<br>sclerometer 硬度计；scleroderma 硬皮病 |
| 软化(softening) | malaci(o)- | malacic 软化的；splenomalacia 脾软化；<br>aortomalacia 主动脉软化；cardiomalacia 心肌软化 |
| 狭窄<br>(narrowing) | sten(o)- | esophagostenosis 食管狭窄；angiostenosis 血管狭窄；<br>enterostenosis 肠道狭窄；cardiostenosis 心腔狭窄 |
| 肿大(dilation) | -ectasis<br>megalo-<br>-megaly | bronchiectasis 支气管扩张；lymphadenectasis 淋巴结肿大；<br>megalocardia 心肥大；hepatomegaly 肝肿大；splenomegaly 脾肿大；<br>hepatolienomegaly 肝脾肿大 |

**Task 10　Learn the prefixes, suffixes or roots in the table by heart and then choose the best answer to finish the exercises.**

1. The Chinese meaning for "melanoma" is _____.

A. 黑色素瘤　　　B. 肌纤维瘤　　　C. 肿瘤细胞　　　D. 致癌基因

2. Fill in the blank with the combining part for the medical term "神经病": neuro-_____?

A. oma　　　B. pathy　　　C. ectasis　　　D. itis

3. The Chinese meaning for "arteriosclerosis" is _____.

A. 硬皮病　　　B. 硬化症　　　C. 动脉硬化症　　　D. 动脉软化症

4. The English term for "脾软化" is _____.

A. arteriosclerosis　　B. cardiomalacia　　C. aortomalacia　　D. splenomalacia

5. The English term for "肠道狭窄" is _____.

A. angiostenosis　　B. cardiostenosis　　C. esophagostenosis　　D. enterostenosis

6. The word which has something to do with "enlargement" is _____.

A. angiostenosis　　B. cardiostenosis　　C. hepatomegaly　　D. enterostenosis

7. To choose a word for "支气管扩张", its correct spelling is _____.

A. bronchitis　　B. bronchiectasis　　C. bronchoscope　　D. bronchopneumonia

8. The following words have the meaning of fever except _____.

A. pathogen　　B. pyrexia　　C. hyperpyrexia　　D. pyretolysis

9. Which word has the meaning of "胆囊切除术"? _____

A. hepatolithiasis　　B. cholecystectomy　　C. cholecystolithiasis　　D. cholecystoctomy

10. The following words have the meaning of "disease" except _____.

A. gastropathy　　B. glucometer　　C. neuropathy　　D. nephropathy

*Note*

# Unit 10　The Reproductive System

## Learning Objectives：

To remember some key English words related to the reproductive system.

To understand the conversation about intravenous injection and talk about the topic.

To read and understand the main ideas and the details of the passages about the reproductive system.

To learn to write an essay with the help of the given sample writing.

To learn by heart some word roots，prefixes and suffixes about the reproductive system.

## Part 1　Look and Learn

**Warming-up 1：Look at the following pictures，talk about them and then finish Task 1.**

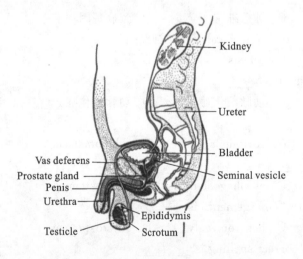

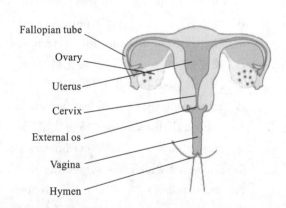

## New Words & Phrases

kidney ['kɪdnɪ] n. 肾脏

ureter [jʊ'riːtər] n. 输尿管

bladder ['blædə(r)] n. 膀胱

seminal vesicle 精囊

gland [glænd] n. 腺

vas deferens 输精管

prostate gland 前列腺

penis ['pi:nɪs] n. 阴茎

urethra [jʊ'ri:θrə] n. 尿道

testicle ['testɪkl] n. 睾丸

epididymis [epɪ'dɪdɪmɪs] n. 附睾

scrotum ['skrəʊtəm] n. 阴囊

fallopian tube 输卵管

ovary ['əʊvərɪ] n. 卵巢

uterus ['ju:tərəs] n. 子宫

cervix ['sɜ:vɪks] n. 子宫颈

external os 宫颈口

vagina [və'dʒaɪnə] n. 阴道

hymen ['haɪmən] n. 处女膜

**Task 1** **Match the words in the left column with the explanations in the right column.**

| 1. kidney | A. either of a pair of thick-walled tubes that carry urine from the kidney to the urinary bladder |
| --- | --- |
| 2. bladder | B. the organ in women and female animals in which babies develop before they are born |
| 3. ovary | C. either of the two organs in the body that remove waste products from the blood and produce urine |
| 4. uterus | D. an organ that is shaped like a bag in which liquid waste (urine) collects before it is passed out of the body |
| 5. ureter | E. either of the two organs in a woman's body that produce eggs |

**Warming-up 2**: **Look at the following pictures about medical instruments, talk about them and then finish Task 2.**

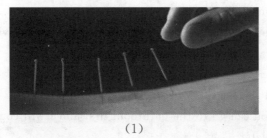

(1)

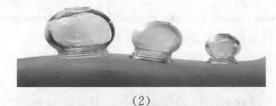

(2)

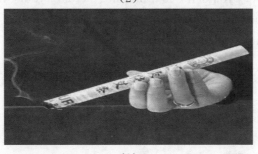

(3)

*Note*

101

## New Words

jar [dʒɑː(r)] n. 罐子

moxa ['mɒksə] n. 艾蒿

filiform [ 'fɪlɪfɔːm] adj. 丝状的

**Task 2　Match the picture number with the proper English and Chinese meaning.**

| Picture number | English | Chinese |
| --- | --- | --- |
| | cupping jar | 火罐 |
| | moxa stick | 艾条 |
| | filiform needle | 毫针 |

# Part 2　Listen and Learn

## Situation Dialogue：Intravenous Therapy

扫码听
对话 1

**Task 3　Listen to the audio episode one and fill in the missing words referring to the original text. Then check your writing against the original.**

Nurse：Morning, Miss Susan. I am Mary. I will be looking after you today.

Patient：Morning, Mary. Pleased to meet you. How does my 1. _____ culture look? I can't handle the pain any more. Today I have to go to 2. _____ more often.

Nurse：Your urine culture indicated that you have a urinary tract 3. _____. And Doctor Wilson prescribed intravenous 4. _____ according to your sensitivity test.

Patient：You mean you will give me an IV right now?

Nurse：Yes, if you are ready.

Patient：OK. Do I need to take the 5. _____ first?

Nurse：No need. But you can go to the bathroom first and I will come back later.

Patient：Sure. See you later.

**Task 4　Listen to the audio episode two and complete the answers according to the questions.**

1. What did the nurse do before giving the patient an IV?

The nurse checked _____ first.

2. What are the steps to have an IV?

Lie down and make yourself comfortable. Hold your hand for a minute. Then _____ your hand.

3. If the patient needs help, what can she do?

Please ring the _____ if the patient needs help.

扫码听
对话 2

*Note*

# Part 3　Read and Learn

**Passage A**

扫码听
课文 A

## Introduction to the Reproductive System

The reproductive system is a collection of internal and external organs — in both males and females — that work together for the purpose of procreating. Due to its vital role in the survival of the species, many scientists argue that the reproductive system is among the most important systems in the entire body.

The male reproductive system consists of two major parts: the testes, where sperm are produced, and the penis. The penis and urethra belong to both the urinary and reproductive systems in males. The testes are carried in an external pouch known as the scrotum, where they normally remain slightly cooler than body temperature to facilitate sperm production.

The major internal organs of the female reproductive system include the vagina and uterus, which act as the receptacle for semen, and the ovaries, which produce the female's ova. The vagina is attached to the uterus through the cervix, while the fallopian tubes connect the uterus to the ovaries. In response to hormonal changes, one ovum, or egg — or more in the case of multiple births — is released and sent down the fallopian tube during ovulation. If not fertilized, this ovum is eliminated as a result of menstruation.

Fertilization occurs if a sperm enters the fallopian tube and burrows into the ovum. While the fertilization usually occurs in the oviducts, it can also happen in the uterus itself. The ovum then becomes implanted in the lining of the uterus, where it begins the processes of embryogenesis (in which the embryo forms) and morphogenesis (in which the fetus begins to take shape). When the fetus is mature enough to survive outside of the womb, the cervix dilates and contractions of the uterus propel it through the birth canal.

## New Words

reproductive [ˌriːprəˈdʌktɪv] adj. 生殖的

procreating [ˈprəʊkrieɪtɪŋ] n. 生育

testes [ˈtestiːz] n. 睾丸

sperm [spɜːm] n. 精子

pouch [paʊtʃ] n. 小袋子

facilitate [fəˈsɪlɪteɪt] v. 促进

receptacle [rɪˈseptəkl] n. 容器

semen [ˈsiːmən] n. 精液

ova [ˈəʊvə] n. 卵子（pl.）ovum 的复数

hormonal [hɔːˈməʊnl] adj. 荷尔蒙的，激素的

ovum [ˈəʊvəm] n. 卵子

ovulation [ˌɒvjuˈleɪʃn] n. 排卵

fertilize [ˈfɜːtəlaɪz] v. 受精

eliminate [ɪˈlɪmɪneɪt] v. 消除

menstruation [ˌmenstruˈeɪʃn] n. 月经

*Note*

burrow ['bʌrəʊ] v. 钻到……里去

oviduct ['əʊvɪdʌkt] adj. 输卵管

embryo ['embriəʊ] n. 胚胎

embryogenesis [ˌembriəʊ'dʒenɪsɪs] n. 胚胎发生（形成）

morphogenesis [ˌmɔrfə'dʒenəsəs] n. 形态发生（形成）

fetus ['fiːtəs] n. 胎儿

womb [wuːm] n. 子宫

dilate [daɪ'leɪt] v. 扩大，(使)膨胀

propel [prə'pel] v. 推动，驱动

**Task 5    Fill in the blanks with the words given below and change the word forms if necessary.**

1. The task of this class session is to discuss the diagnosis and treatment of the upper _____(urine) tract infection.

2. The fetus is propelled out of the birth canal by the _____(contract) of the uterus.

3. The sperm burrows into the egg, and then the fetus implants in the lining of the _____(uterus).

4. A few days later, the newly mother _____(survive) the postpartum complications and hugged her baby the first time.

5. The urethra of the male, different from that of the female, is either a urinary organ and also a _____(reproduction) organ.

6. The _____(hormone) level of the pregnant woman is vital for the development and security of the fetus.

7. The process of _____(fertilize) takes place in the oviducts, and also happens in the uterus.

8. A _____(collect) of the internal and external organs such as uterus, cervix and penis, consists the reproductive system.

9. The jaundice of the newborn baby is _____(slight) better than that yesterday, and will be taken care of in hospital for another 2 days.

10. The female produces only one _____(ova) each month usually, so one pregnancy one baby generally.

**Task 6    Choose the correct answer according to the passage.**

1. Which of the followings is the main content of the passage? _____

A. The function of the reproductive system

B. The organs that consist of the reproductive system

C. The principle of the reproductive system working

D. The difference of the reproductive system between the male and the female

2. Which of the followings is not one of the organs of the female reproductive system? _____

A. uterus          B. ovary          C. cervix          D. sperm

3. Which of the following organs of the male is different from the others? _____

A. urethra          B. penis          C. testes          D. scrotum

4. Where does the fetus develop? _____

A. in the uterus                          B. in the fallopian tubes

C. in the vagina                          D. in the cervix

*Note*

5. Which of the following statements is true according to the passage? _____

A. The fertilization take place in the vagina

B. The fertilization is the process that the embryo forms and develop into fetus

C. The fertilization can occur in the oviduct and the uterus

D. The fertilization can take place in the reproductive system of the male

**Task 7  Arrange the following steps about external chest compression in proper sequence based on the medical procedure.**

_____ Lay the casualty flat on the ground and kneel beside him facing his chest. To find his breastbone (the bone which runs down the centre of the chest), first locate the point where the end of his ribs meet in the middle. This is at the bottom of the breastbone. Measure two finger widths above this junction and place the heel of the other hand above them, keep your fingers off the ribs.

_____ When you reach 15, move back to the casualty's head, tilt the chin back and give him two breaths of mouth-to-mouth.

_____ Cover your hand with the heel of your other hand and lock your fingers together.

_____ Kneel upright so that your shoulders are directly over the casualty's breastbone and your arms are straight. Press down about 4.50 cm, and then release the pressure but do not remove your hands. Complete 15 compressions at a rate of about 80 per minute by counting "one-and-two-and-" as you work.

_____ When you can feel the pulse again, stop pumping immediately. Continue with mouth-to-mouth until natural breathing is restored, and then stop assistance and place the casualty in the recovery position.

_____ Continue giving 15 heart compressions followed by two breaths of mouth-to-mouth. Stop after one minute to check for the pulse; check it again every three minutes.

**Passage B**

### Endometriosis

Endometriosis is defined as the abnormal growth of endometrial cells. The same cells that make up the lining of the uterus shed monthly in the menstrual process. These cells can position themselves in the lower abdomen on areas such as the fallopian tubes and the ovaries. However, unlike uterine cells, they have no passage-way out of the body so they stay where they are and continue their cycle. During menstruation, the normal uterine lining is sloughed off and expelled through the vagina, but transplanted tissue has no means of exiting in the body. The result is internal bleeding, inflammation, and scarring. One of the serious consequences of this scarring is infertility. These growths are generally not malignant or cancerous. But they can rupture and spread to new areas. Dr. Redwine describes the progressive nature of endometriosis lesions as following: "First seen as clear vesicles, then become red, then progress to black lesions over a period of 7-10 years. Water blister lesions become blue dome cysts over a period of 4-10 years. Clear lesions are seen at the average age of 21.5, while black scarred lesions are seen at 31.9 years old. The progression from clear to red to black with age confirms the progressive nature of this disease if left untreated. In 47%-64% of the women, this disease will progress without therapy."

Researchers are looking into a blood test to assist in examining women with symptoms of endometriosis. CA-125 is a cell protein found in pelvic organs that appears to be elevated in cases of moderate or severe endometriosis. An ultrasound device can be indispensable in diagnosing large cysts

扫码听
课文 B

*Note*

and other characteristics of progressing endometriosis. Laparoscopy, when used correctly, usually 100% accurate in diagnosing endometriosis. Diagnosis of endometriosis is generally considered uncertain until proven by laparoscopy. The laparoscopy indicates the location, extent and size of the growths. The cause of endometriosis is an enigma. It is not known why some women suffer from it while others appear to be perfectly healthy. There is the retrograde bleeding theory. This theory implies that retrograde bleeding through the fallopian tubes during menstruation causes endometriosis. Endometriosis is more prevalent in women whose mothers were treated with DES hormone during pregnancy and in women who have pain with their menstruation. The most widely held theory states that endometriosis occurs when endometrial fragments attach to nearby pelvic structures and grow. Endometrial cells are frequently found in peritoneal fluid in all women at the time of menses. One would expect endometriosis to develop in all women. This is not the case. Women with menstrual abnormalities, heavy bleeding or frequent periods, short cycles, early puberty, are more likely to get endometriosis. Another theory indicates that hormonal problems allow this tissue to take root and grow in women who develop endometriosis.

Endometriosis is categorized and diagnosed in four stages based on locations affected. Stage 1, or minimal disease: superficial and filmy adhesions. Stage 2, or mild disease: superficial and deep endometriosis, filmy adhesions. Stage 3, or moderate disease: superficial and deep endometriosis, filmy and dense adhesions. Stage 4, or severe disease: superficial and deep endometriosis, dense adhesions. Even though the stages may seem similar, the sizes and number of areas diseased indicate diagnosis. It would seem that these symptoms should help to ensure a proper diagnosis, but there could be different reasons for the discomforts other than endometriosis. It is also important to note that not all women with the disease suffer from symptoms, even in Stage 4. Even though some women with endometriosis are asymptomatic, pain plays a large role in a significant percentage of women with the disease. Pain was reported to interfere in some way with all aspects of activities of daily living. Seventy-eight percent were interfered with sleep, which was significant because fatigue tends to accelerate the severity of pain. Pain reported by 100% 1-2 days prior to cycle, 71% mid-cycle, 47% other times, 40% pain throughout, and 7% intermittent pain with no pattern. Since the onset of pain, 81% reported pain was progressive. Women were asked to describe their moods and feelings when experiencing pain. 84% reported feeling depressed, 75% irritable, 63% experienced mood swings, 54% feeling anxious, 53% angry, 51% negative, 43% helpless, 35% fearful and powerless, 32% worried, 31% insecure, and 19% hopeless. Although hormonal treatments may be somewhat effective in relieving symptoms, all of them can have unpleasant side effect.

## New Words

endometriosis [ˈendəʊˌmiːtrɪˈəʊsɪs] n. 子宫内膜异位症

shed [ʃed] v. 流出

slough [slʌf] v. 脱落

malignant [məˈlɪgnənt] adj. 恶性的

cancerous [ˈkænsərəs] adj. 癌的

lesion [ˈliːʒən] n. 损伤

vesicle [ˈvesɪkl] n. 泡，囊

blister [ˈblɪstə] n. 水疱

dome [dəʊm] n. 穹顶，圆顶

cyst [sɪst] n. 囊，包囊

indispensable [ˌɪndɪˈspensəbl] adj. 不可或缺的,必不可少的

laparoscopy [ˌlæpəˈrɒskəpɪ] n. 腹腔镜检查

enigma [ɪˈnɪgmə] n. 费解的事物,令人困惑的处境

retrograde [ˈretrəʊgreɪd] adj. 倒退的,退化的

peritoneal [ˌperɪtəˈniːəl] adj. 腹膜的

menses [ˈmensiːz] n. 月经

puberty [ˈpjuːbətɪ] n. 青春期

filmy [ˈfɪlmɪ] adj. 薄薄的

adhesion [ədˈhiːʒən] n. 粘连

asymptomatic [ˌeɪsɪmptəˈmætɪk] adj. 无症状的

intermittent [ˌɪntəˈmɪtənt] adj. 断断续续的

## Exercises

**Task 8    Match the words or phrases with similar meaning in the two columns.**

|  | A |  | B |
|---|---|---|---|
| 1. | uterus | a. | suggest |
| 2. | imply | b. | monthly bleeding |
| 3. | therapy | c. | no symptoms |
| 4. | menses | d. | rose |
| 5. | cyst | e. | cancerous |
| 6. | elevated | f. | damage |
| 7. | malignant | g. | not pregnant |
| 8. | lesion | h. | womb |
| 9. | infertility | i. | treatment |
| 10. | asymptomatic | j. | bladder |

**Task 9    Choose the right answer to fill in the blanks in the passage.**

It was Sunday. I had one last patient to see. I approached her ward in a hurry and stood at the doorway. She was an older woman, ___1___ to put socks on her swollen feet. I spoke quickly to the nurse, scanned her chart noting she was in ___2___ condition. I was almost in the clear.

She asked if I could help put on her socks. Instead, I launched into a monologue: "How are you feeling? The nurse mentioned you're ___3___ to see your son who's visiting you today..."

She stopped me. "Sit down, doctor. This is my story, not your story."

I was surprised and ___4___. I sat down. I helped her with the socks and she told me that her only son lived around the corner from her, but she had not seen him in five years. She believed that this contributed ___5___ to her health problems. I asked if there was anything else I could do for her. She shook her head ___6___ and smiled. All she wanted me to do was to listen.

Listening to someone's story ___7___ less than expensive diagnostic testing but is the key to healing and diagnosis.

I often thought of what that woman taught me and ___8___ myself of the importance of stopping, sitting down, and truly listening.

Twenty years later, I still teach med students and tell them I believe in the power of ___9___. I tell them I know first-hand that ___10___ healing takes place within me when someone stops, sits down, and listens to my story.

*Note*

107

1. A. struggle        B. struggles       C. and struggle    D. struggling
2. A. stable          B. bad             C. well            D. worse
3. A. worry           B. hurry           C. anxious         D. worrying
4. A. shy             B. embarrassed     C. anxious         D. nervous
5. A. a little        B. greatly         C. badly           D. slightly
6. A. no              B. not             C. none            D. neither
7. A. takes           B. pays            C. costs           D. gives
8. A. remained        B. reminded        C. retained        D. maintained
9. A. talking         B. telling         C. visiting        D. listening
10. A. measurable     B. immeasurable    C. valuable        D. invaluable

# Part 4    Write and Learn

### Essay Writing (2)

**Direction: Read the following writing sample carefully. Design and finish an imitated writing task with similar style.**

解决问题类议论文常为三段：第一段，简明扼要地点明要论述的话题，并说明其危害；第二段，中心段，主要分析造成该问题的原因；第三段，结尾段，提出解决的办法。

【Sample】

Reduce the Traffic Accident

Outline：1. 近年来，交通事故的发生率呈上升趋势。

2. 交通事故增加的主要原因。

3. 采用相应的措施减少事故。

With the development of society, a growing number of people can afford private cars. Meanwhile, road accidents are often reported in our country and it is amazing that road accidents cause too many deaths, injuries and millions of losses.

Perhaps the key reasons of road accidents are as follows. First, among those accidents, driver's carelessness and lack of the awareness of safety are responsible for most of them. Driving after drinking alcohol, speeding and overloading are the common mistakes that drivers are likely to commit. Second, some people fail to observe traffic regulations. They either cross the street with red-light or step on the wrong lane instead of on sidewalks. Last, some roads are in a poor condition. What's worse, there are no traffic signals on some roads.

It is high time we do something to cut the road accidents. On the one hand, people need to be educated to observe the traffic rules. On the other hand, the government should take effective measures, such as "one-way street" or "no left-turn" at certain crossroads to regulate traffic movements. Only in these ways, it is possible to reduce the road accidents in the future.

【Assignment】

Old Men's Problem

Outline：1. 越来越多的老年人独居。

2. 老年人独居的困难（生活、经济、情感等）。

3. 如何解决老年人的问题？

# Part 5    Prefixes, Suffixes & Roots

**Reproductive System（生殖系统）**

| 汉语（英语） | 常用词根 | 例    词 |
|---|---|---|
| 生殖（reproduction） | genit(o)- | genital 生殖的；urogenital 泌尿生殖的 |
| 子宫（womb） | uter(o)-；hyster(o)-；metr(o)- | uterine 子宫的；extrauterine 子宫外的；hysterotomy 子宫切开术；perimetrium 子宫外膜 |
| 膀胱（bladder） | vesic(o)-；cyst(o)- | vesical 膀胱的；rectovesical 直肠膀胱的；cystitis 膀胱炎；cystostomy 膀胱造瘘术 |
| 阴道（vagina） | vagin(o)-；colp(o)- | vaginitis 阴道炎；colposcopy 阴道镜检查；colpoperineoplasty 阴道会阴成形术 |
| 月经（menstruation） | men(o)- | menopause 绝经；amenorrhea 闭经 |
| 胚胎（embryo） | embry(o)- | embryology 胚胎学；tubalembryo 胚胎输卵管 |
| 羊膜，羊水（amnion） | amni(o)- | amniotic 羊膜的；amniocentesis 羊膜穿刺术；amnioscopy 羊膜镜检查 |
| 胎盘（placenta） | placent(o)- | placental 胎盘的；uteroplacental 子宫胎盘的 |
| 胎儿（fetus） | fet(o)- | fetal 胎儿的；fetocardiogram 胎儿心动图 |
| 产次（parity） | -para | primipara 初产妇；multipara 多产妇 |
| 卵泡（follicle） | follicul(o)- | follicular 卵泡的；folliculosis 滤泡增殖 |
| 卵巢（ovary） | ovari(o)- | ovariotomy 卵巢切除术；ovariotubal 卵巢输卵管的 |
| 精子（semen） | semin(o)- | seminal 精液的；insemination 受精 |
| 阴囊（scrotum） | scrot(o)- | scrotitis 阴囊炎；scrotectomy 阴囊切除术 |
| 阴茎（penis） | pen(o)-；phall(o)- | penitis 阴茎炎；phallalgia 阴茎痛 |

**Task 10    Learn the prefixes, suffixes or roots in the table by heart and then choose the best answer to finish the exercises.**

1. The Chinese meaning for the word "genital" is _____.

A. 生殖            B. 泌尿生殖的          C. 生殖的              D. 生殖器

2. The correct medical term for "阴道炎" is _____.

A. vulvitis          B. vulvovaginitis      C. vulvaginiti        D. vaginitis

3. "子宫切开术" is called as _____.

A. hysterotomy        B. uterotomy        C. metrotomy          D. wombotomy

4. The correct interpretation of the word "amenorrhea" is _____.

A. 月经            B. 绝经              C. 闭经                D. 月经不调

5. The correct spelling of the word for Chinese "羊膜" is _____.

A. amino            B. amnion            C. ammino            D. annion

6. Fill in the blank with the combining part for the medical term "羊膜穿刺术": _____-centesis.

A. amnio      B. amnion      C. ammio      D. annio

7. The correct interpretation of the word "scrotitis " is _____.

A. 阴茎痛      B. 阴茎炎      C. 阴囊炎      D. 阴囊肿大

8. The correct Chinese equivalent for the word "tubalembryo" is _____.

A. 胚胎学      B. 胚胎      C. 输卵管      D. 胚胎输卵管

9. The woman delivering the baby for the first time is called as _____.

A. deutiapara      B. nullipara      C. primipara      D. multipara

10. The correct spelling form for the word "胎儿心动图" is _____.

A. fetocardiogram          B. fetal cardiogram

C. fetus cardiogram         D. embryo cardiogram

# Final Review

## I Listening

### Part 1

**Questions 1-5**

- You will hear five extracts from conversations taking place in different clinical departments.
- For questions 1-5, choose letter A-F the case each doctor is discussing.
- You will hear each extracts twice.

扫码听
短文

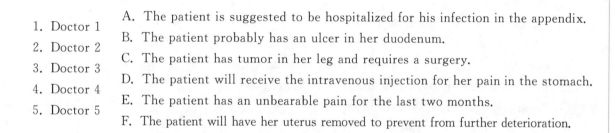

1. Doctor 1    A. The patient is suggested to be hospitalized for his infection in the appendix.

2. Doctor 2    B. The patient probably has an ulcer in her duodenum.

3. Doctor 3    C. The patient has tumor in her leg and requires a surgery.

4. Doctor 4    D. The patient will receive the intravenous injection for her pain in the stomach.

5. Doctor 5    E. The patient has an unbearable pain for the last two months.

               F. The patient will have her uterus removed to prevent from further deterioration.

### Part 2

**Questions 6-10**

- You will hear a passage about heart rhythm and heart failure.
- For questions 6-10, choose the right answer.
- You will hear the passage twice.

扫码听
短文

6. 75 beats per minute is the normal resting heart rate. _____

A. right          B. wrong          C. not mentioned

7. In arrhythmia, there may be early beats. _____

A. right          B. wrong          C. not mentioned

8. Heart failure occurs when the heart maintains sufficient cardiac output. _____

A. right          B. wrong          C. not mentioned

9. Heart failure can only occur in the left side of the heart. _____

A. right          B. wrong          C. not mentioned

10. The symptom of right heart failure is swelling. _____

A. right          B. wrong          C. not mentioned

*Note*

**Part 3**

**Questions 11-15**

• You will hear an interview about AIDS.

• For questions 11-15, choose the best answer.

• You will hear the interview twice.

11. AIDS is a term used for HIV infection in its _____.

A. most advanced stages

B. most initial stages

C. stages at any level

12. Without treatment, most people infected with HIV would develop signs _____.

A. in a varied length of time

B. within 5-10 years

C. between 10-15 years

13. The most common life-threatening infection affecting HIV/AIDS patients is _____.

A. nephritis

B. sepsis

C. tuberculosis

14. Which is not a benefit of an HIV test? _____

A. access treatment, care and support to prolong life

B. see a doctor earlier to find a way to cure HIV infection

C. take measures to prevent the spread of HIV to others

15. Good and continue HIV treatment could _____.

A. cure HIV infection at an early stage

B. slow the deterioration of HIV infection

C. promote life expectancy and creativity

## Ⅱ Reading and Writing

**Part 1**

**Questions 1-7**

• Read the following conversation about IV infusion.

• Complete these extracts from the nurse's instructions using the verbs in the box.

Jane: All right, Emile. Let's get the next IV bag ready. Before we start, we need to wash our hands.

Emile: Oh, right. Of course.

Jane: OK, now we can start. First, we'll check the IV solution against the IV prescription.

Emile: OK. The prescription is for 5% dextrose.

Jane: That's it. Here is the IV infusion. Can you check it with me? This is a bag of 5% dextrose.

Emile: Yes, I can see the label, 5% dextrose.

Jane: Next, I'm going to prime the line. To prime the line, you run the IV fluid through the IV tubing of the giving set.

Emile: The giving set has one end to go into the IV bag and the other end is for connection to the patient's cannula. Is that right?

Jane: That's right. We are going to run this IV infusion through an IV infusion pump. Next we need to set the rate on the infusion pump. What's the rate, Emile?

Emile: The rate is 125 milliliters per hour.

Jane: That's right. It's an 8-hour litre. After that, I'll start the infusion pump.

Jane: Yes, it is. OK, that's ready. Now, I'll connect the IV to patient's cannula. Then, I'll start the infusion pump.

Jane: Now we both have to sign the IV prescription.

Emile: OK, here?

Jane: That's right. The last thing is to write up the fluid balance chart.

Emile: OK, I think I have all that.

Jane: Let's go over it again. Can you tell me the seven steps we went through?

> check  connect  prime  set  sign  start  write up

First we need to wash our hands.

We'll 1. _____ the IV solution against the IV prescription.

I'm going to 2. _____ the line.

3. _____ the rate on the infusion pump.

I'll 4. _____ the IV to the patient's cannula.

I'll 5. _____ the infusion pump.

We have to 6. _____ the IV prescription.

The last thing is to 7. _____ the fluid balance chart.

### Part 2

### Questions 1-5

• Read the following passage on the immune system and health of gut bacteria. Five sentences have been removed from the passage.

• Choose from sentences A-F the one which best fits each blank 1-5. There is one more extra sentence which you do not need to use.

#### Immune system and health of gut bacteria

The gastrointestinal(GI) tract is very important in a person's health. Most people think of heart or lungs first as being the most vital organs, which they are, but without being able to eat, poop or absorb nutrients, our body wouldn't work properly.

1. _____. Not only does it hold all of our food and drinks, but it is able to contract and relax, creating chyme that will be sent to the duodenum and small intestine. Through a complex system of glands, blood flow, the stomach secretes 1,500 to 3,000 ml of gastric juices daily, adjusting to the different foods we ingest.

These juices come from several glands within the gastric mucosa, cardiac glands, chief cells, mucus and endocrine. 2. _____. The emptying process alone involve neural impulses, hormones secreted by the small intestine, and chyme. If any of the steps is interrupted, the patient develops health problems.

It has been thought for a long time that the immune system is linked to the bacteria in the gut; now there is research to prove it. The article "Immune System Affects Gut Bacteria Evolution" by Instituto Gulbenkian states, "Our health is strongly dependent on the diversity of bacteria that inhabits our intestinal tract and on how the immune system tolerates it or responds to the pathogenic bacteria to prevent disease." 3. _____. This finding is especially useful in patients with

*Note*

inflammatory bowel disease, suggesting that a custom treatment is needed.

The lead research, Isabel Gordo and Jocelyne Demengeot are the first to show the link between the immune system and gut bacteria. Their research focused on *Escherichia coli* which is the first bacteria to colonize in newborn. While in mice with the healthy immune systems, the growth of bacteria was predictable. 4._____.

The immune system can regulate the microbes in the gut. When that goes wrong, there is no way to predict what is going to happen to the bacteria in the gut which leads to the understanding that treating those with IBD(a group of diseases causing chronic inflammation in the colon) on an individual basis rather than a blanket therapy will be the new standard of care.

Medicine makes new strides daily, new procedures, research, medications that help patients live a healthier life. 5._____ . Those of us who work in the GI labs know how important eating, digesting, absorbing minerals and vitamins, and of course pooping is to our patients. If a patient cannot eat, they lose weight along with their natural defense to fight diseases. We see how miserable they are when suffering from reflux, constipation, IBD, and hundreds of other disorder of the GI tract.

A. Each of those glands/cells work together to break down the food we eat into chyme that is then dumped into the duodenum

B. The two main IBD's ones are Crohn's desease and ulcerative colitis, both of which present with diarrhea, abdominal pain and cramps

C. When a person's immune system is depressed, correspondingly, the gut bacteria changes creating a domino effect on the host's decreasing health

D. This exciting new information proves that our health depends on what our gut and GI tract are doing

E. In those lacking lymphocytes(white blood cells, very important in the immune system), there was an unpredictable variation

F. The gut is an amazing part of the GI tract, digesting food, getting nutrients ready for the body to absorb and send them to where they need to be

**Part 3**
**Questions 1-10**

• Read the following passage.

• Choose the most appropriate words to fill in the blanks from the choices(A ,B, or C) given below.

### A Mistake I Made in a Clinical

Hi there, senior nursing student here. The other day I had my 1._____ day of clinical in the PICU and I made a completely stupid and dangerous mistake. My poor patient was on numerous drips and have numerous IVs in her right arm. One of the IVs went bad over night 2._____, and another went bad soon after we completed our morning assessment. She really needed 3._____ IV and she was a very hard stick. After about 30 minutes of trying, the vascular access team finally got an IV on her. Shortly after, we get busy by the doctors rounding, linen changes, trach suctioning, etc. The nurse then asks me if I can 4._____ the IV that had gone bad upon our morning assessment. So I go ahead and take out the IV. It was the wrong IV. I 5._____ took out the brand new IV that they had just placed! Now the two IVs were very close to each other, both on the right forearm. However I still should know which was which considering I had watched them place the IV not even an hour ago. So basically I felt absolutely 6. _____ and incompetent for the rest of the day. And worse, I will be working with this same nurse for the next month. I feel like I could write a book titled "How to make your preceptor hate you 101". Oh and even worse, this is the unit that I would like to be hired into when I 7. _____ in 6 months. The nurse continually told me 8. _____ the day not to feel bad, that it wasn't that big of a deal, but I know it was. This patient was a critically ill patient. She needed that IV access. Thankfully they were able to place a midline in her later on that day, but still. It was completely my fault that they had to do that. I guess now I am asking for advice on how to mentally move past this, and on how to make it up to my preceptor. Are any hopes of becoming a PICU nurse completely ruined? I am trying to let it go and go into my next shift with a 9. _____ attitude, but I just feel like I have 10. _____ the whole thing by this one mistake. Any comments or advice would be greatly appreciated.

1. A. first            B. last            C. second
2. A. class            B. work            C. shift
3. A. the              B. another         C. one
4. A. take out         B. take on         C. take off
5. A. immediately      B. accidentally    C. reluctantly
6. A. good             B. terrible        C. happy
7. A. graduate         B. come            C. leave
8. A. that             B. throughout      C. /
9. A. positive         B. negative        C. neutral
10. A. destroy         B. done            C. ruined

**Part 4**

Write an essay of about 150 words on the topic of "Hospice Care". You should base your essay on the clues given below.

1. What is hospice care?
2. Your opinions about hospice care.

*Note*

115

# Appendix A　Transcripts of Dialogues

## Unit 1

### Dialogue 1　Receiving a Patient (1)

Doctor: Good morning. I am Doctor Sterling. How can I help you?

Patient: Good morning, Doctor. I am Emily. I have a fever and sore throat since yesterday.

Doctor: Oh, did you take your temperature?

Patient: Yes, I did. The highest temperature was 39.8 ℃ at 11:00 pm last night. I took one pill of aspirin and feel much better.

Doctor: Any other symptoms?

Patient: I have a runny nose and headache, too.

Doctor: OK, let me take your temperature first. Please keep this thermometer under your armpit for 5 minutes. Open your mouth and say "Ah", please. Your tonsils and larynx are red and swollen. Your temperature is 38.5 ℃. Your breathing sounds are normal and there is no problem with your lungs. You'd better take the blood test, OK? This paper is for the lab test.

Patient: Sure. I really hope I get better as soon as possible. See you later.

(to be continued)

### New Words & Phrases

sore adj. 疼痛的

sore throat 咽喉痛

aspirin n. 阿司匹林

thermometer n. 温度计,体温表

tonsil n. 扁桃体

larynx n. 咽喉

blood test 血液检查

### Dialogue 2　Receiving a Patient (2)

(30 minutes later, the patient comes back)

Patient: Excuse me, doctor. Here's the result of my blood test.

Doctor: OK. The blood routine shows that your WBC is 12,000/mm³, N 80%, L 20%. It indicates that you have an upper respiratory tract infection. Are you allergic to any drugs or foods?

Patient: No. I don't think so.

Doctor: I'll prescribe amoxicillin for you. It's an oral medicine. Take 2 tablets 3 times a day

116

around the clock. You can take aspirin if fever persists. You'd better take vitamin C, 2 tablets 3 times a day, too. And drink a lot of liquids and have plenty of rest.

Patient: How long should I take the medicine?

Doctor: Take it for 5 days, and come back for a follow-up check up. Don't hesitate to call me if you have any problem.

Patient: Thank you so much. I really appreciate your help.

## New Words & Phrases

blood routine 血常规

WBC (abbr. white blood cell count) 白细胞计数

upper respiratory tract infection 上呼吸道感染

allergic adj. 过敏的

amoxicillin n. 阿莫西林

follow-up n.（对患者的）随访

# Unit 2

### Dialogue 3　Consulting a Doctor(1)

Doctor: Hi, I am Doctor Susan. How can I help you?

Patient: Hi, doctor. I am Mary. Would you please take a look at my lab result?

Doctor: Sure. Take a seat please.

Patient: Thank you. This is the blood result of my kidney function, and the other is the liver function.

Doctor: I see. I'd like to know your medical history first. Have you had any problem with your kidney or liver?

Patient: Yes. I was told I have IgA nephropathy 5 years ago because both my uric acid and creatinine levels were too high. My urine has been tea-colored for almost 5 years.

Doctor: Did you have a biopsy?

Patient: No. The doctor suggested the biopsy but I am really afraid of that. So they haven't been able to diagnose the IgA until now.

Doctor: What kind of symptoms do you have now?

Patient: Oh, I have had a gout for a week, and my left foot is still painful and swollen.

(to be continued)

## New Words & Phrases

lab result 实验室检查结果

kidney function 肾功能

liver function 肝功能

IgA(abbr. immunoglobulin A) nephropathy 免疫球蛋白 A 肾病

urine acid 尿酸

creatinine n. 肌酐

biopsy n.（活组织）切片检查法

gout n. 痛风

### Dialogue 4  Consulting a Doctor(2)

Doctor：May I take a look of your foot? Ah, I see. Are you taking any medication?

Patient：Yes. I am taking a painkiller for my gout these days. But I don't remember the name of the medication.

Doctor：Your present lab results are good, and the levels of urine acid and creatinine are normal. You'd better avoid the painkillers since they affect kidney function.

Patient：Good. Your instructions are really helpful. Do I need any other medication for my gout?

Doctor：You could try some Chinese traditional herbs, such as notoginseng, to enhance your blood circulation.

Patient：Oh, really? I haven't heard that before. But I have heard that Chinese traditional medicine does cure some sicknesses. I'd like to try.

Doctor：OK, you can buy some from the drug store.

Patient：Thank you so much. I really appreciate your instructions. Have a good day!

Doctor：You're welcome. Have a good day.

## New Words & Phrases

painkiller n. 止痛药

herb n. 中草药

notoginseng n. 三七

enhance v. 提高,增强

blood circulation 血液循环

# Unit 3

### Dialogue 5  Admitting a Patient(1)

Nurse：Good morning, Mrs. Wilson. I am the nurse of the GI department. My name is Emily. I'll be admitting you to the ward today.

Patient：Good morning, Emily. What should I do now?

Nurse：Would you please come with me to the nurses' office so I can finish the paperwork first?

Patient：Sure. May I sit down?

Nurse：Yes, of course. Please sit down and make yourself comfortable, OK? Can you tell me your full name and your date of birth?

Patient：My full name is Rose Wilson. And I was born on Nov. 15th, 1968.

Nurse：Can you tell me why you are here today?

Patient：Well, um. I've had a duodenal ulcer for about five years. My stools have been black for the past two days. I feel weak, too. My occult blood test is positive, so my doctor suggested for me to come here.

(to be continued)

## New Words & Phrases

admit v. 许可进入,承认

GI (abbr. gastrointestinal) adj. 胃肠的

duodenal adj. 十二指肠的

ulcer n. 溃疡

stool n. 大便

admit a patient 收患者入院

GI department 消化科

### Dialogue 6    Admitting a Patient(2)

Nurse: OK. Would you please give me your past results, such as the barium X rays and gastrointestinal endoscopy? We need to make a copy and put it into your chart.

Patient: Sure. I'll give them to you later.

Nurse: By the way, I'd like to know your past medical history. Have you had any serious illness in the past except the duodenal ulcer?

Patient: No. I think that my duodenal ulcer came from too much pressure in my job. I am busy with my work every day, so I can't take good care of myself.

Nurse: Mm, that's reasonable. I'll take the BP for you now. I'd like you to sit a little closer to this desk and roll up your sleeve. OK, it's one ten over 70, that's good. I'd also like to take your pulse rate.

Patient: Is my pulse too fast? I always feel palpitations these days.

Nurse: Mm, a little bit fast. It's one fifteen. And please put this thermometer under your tongue. You can take it out when you hear the beep. OK, it's 37.0 ℃. Thank you very much for your cooperation, Mrs. Wilson. Now please follow me, and I will show you around the ward.

## New Words & Phrases

Barium n. 钡

endoscopy n. 内镜检查

chart n. 病历

palpitation n. 心悸

ward n. 病房,病区

barium X rays X线钡餐检查

BP (abbr. blood pressure) 血压

gastrointestinal endoscopy 胃肠道内镜检查

pulse rate 脉率

# Unit 4

### Dialogue 7    In the Nurses' Office (1)

Doctor: Hello. Mary, are you looking after Mr. John today?

Nurse: Yes. Any questions?

Doctor: Oh, can we take a few minutes to talk about his situation?

Nurse: Sure. Have a seat, please.

Doctor: Thank you. He was back from the OR an hour ago and there are a lot of orders for him. Let's make sure they are clear.

Nurse：OK. Let me see. Blood pressure, pulse rate and breathing rate every 30 minutes, temperature every 4 hours. And monitor the GCS every 4 hours.

Doctor：And also monitor his I & O, OK?

Nurse：Sure. How about his fluids?

Doctor：Now his potassium levels are very low according to his blood result. Would you please give him a liter of normal saline with 20 millimoles of KCl?

Nurse：Sure. Please fill out the patient's chart first.

(to be continued)

## New Words & Phrases

order n. 医嘱

liter n. 升

potassium n. 钾

millimole n. 毫摩尔

OR (abbr. operation room) 手术室

GCS (abbr. Glasgow Coma Scale) n. 格拉斯哥昏迷评分量表

I & O (abbr. intake and output) 出入量

normal saline 生理盐水

### Dialogue 8　In the Nurses' Office (2)

Doctor：No problem. Thanks for your reminder. The normal saline with 20 millimoles of KCl should be given over 4 hours, OK?

Nurse：I see. Any other fluids?

Doctor：Yes. I will prescribe some antibiotics for him. I'd prefer you to run them through a secondary line(第二条静脉通路).

Nurse：OK. May I run them through the cannula?

Doctor：Right. Make sure the cannula is still working because we didn't use it yesterday. And I want to give him some nutrients with the fluids. These nutrients are sticky, so you can't run them through the cannula in case of blockage.

Nurse：I understand.

Doctor：Furthermore, start him on some oxygen at 2 liters per minute for 3 hours because his oxygen saturation is 90. We also need to monitor his oxygen saturation, OK?

Nurse：Of course. Don't forget to fill out all these orders, doctor.

## New Words & Phrases

fluid n. 液体

antibiotic n. 抗生素

cannula n. 导管,套管

blockage n. 堵塞

nutrient n. 营养物，营养品

saturation n. 饱和度

oxygen saturation 血氧饱和度

# Unit 5

### Dialogue 9    Administering Medications (1)

Nurse: Hi, Janice. Good to see you again.

Patient: Thank you and me too. You look so nice today.

Nurse: How are you doing today?

Patient: Not good, I have a headache and feel dizzy today. My blood pressure was one eighty over one ten (180/110) this morning. That's really high, isn't it?

Nurse: Oh, I see. That's the reason why Dr. Peter prescribed two new medications for you. One is metoprolol, to lower your BP. And another is Lasix, a diuretic.

Patient: Oh, I can't remember the names. Would you please repeat them?

Nurse: Sure, and I'll tell more about them. Metoprolol is in the green box, and I already wrote down the instructions for you. You take this 2 pills once, twice a day, that's 8:00 am before your breakfast and 8:00 pm before your bedtime. Got it?

Patient: Mm, but I have a very poor memory. Instructions on the box are good for me.

(to be continued)

## New Words & Phrases

dizzy adj. 头晕眼花的,眩晕的

diuretic n. 利尿剂

metoprolol n. 美托洛尔

Lasix n. 速尿(呋喃苯胺酸制剂的商品名)

### Dialogue 10    Administering Medications (2)

Nurse: OK, let's continue. You have to put this medication in a cool place because it would be melt at 45 ℃. Another one, Lasix, is in the white box. It's a diuretic (water pill) that prevents your body from absorbing too much salt, allowing the salt to instead be eliminated through the urine. This medication is also used to treat hypertension.

Patient: Does that mean I will pass more urine after I take this medication?

Nurse: Yes, absolutely. The frequency and amount of your urine will be increased. But don't worry, that's the normal effect of the medication. Please let us know if you aren't comfortable or have any problem, OK?

Patient: Thank you. Any other instructions?

Nurse: Oh, by the way, you'd better eat the low-cholesterol, low-fat and low-sodium diet with more dietary fiber. That means that you'd better eat more fresh vegetables and fruits, less salt and meat. That's good for both your hypertension and heart.

Patient: That's really very hard for me. Anyway, I'll try my best to follow your guidance. You are a great nurse.

## New Words & Phrases

urine n. 尿

hypertension n. 高血压

cholesterol n. 胆固醇

fat n. 脂肪

sodium n. 钠

dietary adj. 与饮食有关的，饮食的

fiber n. 纤维

# Transcripts for Midterm Review

**Part 1**

Conversation 1

Nurse (woman)：Are you all right，Mr. Connolly?

Patient (man)：No. I've got a really bad toothache.

Nurse (woman)：Sit down and I'll have a look.

Patient (man)：Thanks.


Conversation 2

Nurse (woman)：How are you feeling，Mr. Jameson?

Patient (man)：Not very well. Can I have some painkillers，please?

Nurse (woman)：Sure. Where does it hurt?

Patient (man)：My upper back is really aching.

Nurse (woman)：OK，I'll get the tablets and a heat pack，too.


Conversation 3

Nurse (woman)：Hello, Jack. How do you feel today?

Patient (man)：Well，my knee really hurts.

Nurse (woman)：Put your leg on this pillow and I'll get you some pain relief for that.

Patient (man)：Thanks，it's really painful. Can I have a ice pack too，please?

Nurse (woman)：Sure. I'll get some for you.


Conversation 4

Nurse (man)：So，what brings you here today，Mrs. Swift?

Patient (woman)：Um, I've been having these really bad headaches.

Nurse (man)：Go on...

Patient (woman)：Well，I keep getting them.

Nurse (man)：Ah-huh? Can you describe them?

Patient (woman)：Um, it's quite a dull pain, but there's a constant throbbing pain as well. It builds up.

Nurse (man)：Mm. Whereabouts do you get these headaches?

Patient (woman)：Here，around the front，around the forehead.


Conversation 5

Nurse (woman)：Good morning，Mr. Douglas. What can I do for you?

Patient (man): I've been having some problems with my breathing.

Nurse (woman): Mm-hmm. Can you tell me a little bit more about it?

Patient (man): Well, I keep getting breathlessness and wheezing in my chest. It all started about two weeks ago, and I've been coughing a lot with it. I thought that it might be a cold, but I found it more and more difficult to catch my breath.

Nurse (woman): Right, so you've had the wheezing and the breathlessness for roughly two weeks.

Patient (man): Yes.

## Part 2

Nurse: Hello, Mrs. Samira? Can you open your eyes, please?

Patient: Ugh.

Nurse: That's it. I'll just take off your oxygen mask. Do you know where you are?

Patient: Hospital.

Nurse: That's right. You've had your operation. How do you feel?

Patient: Cold.

Nurse: That's quite normal after an operation. I'll get you a blanket.

Patient: Mm.

Nurse: There you are. Are you warmer now?

Patient: Er, yes.

Nurse: Are you in any pain?

Patient: Em... no.

Nurse: That's good. You had a painkiller before you left the operation theatre.

Patient: Mm.

Nurse: Do you feel sick the moment?

Patient: No.

Nurse: OK. Some people feel sick after the anaesthetic. All right, I'm just going to take your obs. again.

Patient: OK.

## Part 3

Nurse 1: Hello, Emile. I just took Annabel's 10:00 am Obs. for you.

Nurse 2: Oh, thank you. What were they?

Nurse 1: Her temp is 36.5 ℃ now.

Nurse 2: Oh, that's good.

Nurse 1: Mm, her pulse is 64. BP is one hundred and ten over seventy.

Nurse 2: OK. Pulse 64, BP is one hundred and ten over seventy. How about her resps?

Nurse 1: Oh, it's still 18. Oxygen sats are 98%.

Nurse 2: What about her weight?

Nurse 1: Er... It's 60 kilos. I've charted the Obs. for you.

Nurse 2: Thanks a lot.

*Note*

# Unit 6

### Dialogue 11    Preoperative Nursing (1)

Nurse：Morning, Mr. Peter. I am Cathy. Did you sleep well last night?

Patient：Morning, Cathy. I was a little nervous about the surgery, so I didn't sleep that well.

Nurse：Yes, it's hard for everyone at this point. Do you have any questions about the surgery?

Patient：Mm, I signed the consent form two days ago, and I saw the risks of the operation in the form, such as the complications from the anesthesia, the bleeding, and even death. I am a little afraid of these things.

Nurse (smiles and touches the patient's hand)：I understand it's not easy for you. Actually the consent form tells us all kinds of the possibilities during the surgery, but these risks are very small and not likely to happen to you. It's just standard hospital procedure.

Patient：I see. I hope my surgery is successful. Especially my child is only five years old.

Nurse (smiles)：It will be fine. You should trust the doctors. And you have been on a low-residue diet for three days, right?

Patient：Yes. May I eat today?

Nurse：Yes, but only clear fluids for today. Then you'll start NPO after midnight.

(to be continued)

## New Words & Phrases

preoperative adj. 手术前的

consent form 知情同意书

anesthesia n. 麻醉

bleeding n. 出血

low-residue diet 少渣饮食

NPO (abbr. nothing per mouth) 禁食

### Dialogue 12    Preoperative Nursing (2)

Patient：Does that mean I won't be able to eat or drink anything after midnight?

Nurse：No, you won't. And you will be given an enema tonight around 8：00 pm.

Patient：For what? Is it painful?

Nurse：The enema causes you to have a bowel movement and then lower the risk of contamination from the bowel contents. It won't be painful. I am sure you can handle it.

Patient：OK. If I have to, I will.

Nurse：There are two more things before the surgery. Tomorrow morning you'll be given a nasogastric tube to keep the stomach empty. You'll keep the tube for a few days for gastric decompression. It will also lower the pressure of the incision.

Patient：Oh, my goodness! I hope that's all.

Nurse：It's good for you to know all the details of your procedure. The other tube you'll have is an indwelling catheter, which can be taken out when you can void by yourself. I'll take care of you before and after the operation tomorrow. You'll be just fine.

*Note*

## New Words & Phrases

enema n. 灌肠

bowel n. 肠

bowel movement 大便

contamination n. 污染

nasogastric tube 鼻胃管

decompression n. 减压

incision n. 切口

indwelling catheter 留置尿管

void v. 排空

# Unit 7

### Dialogue 13　Postoperative Nursing Discussion(1)

Head nurse：Hello, everyone. Let's start with Mrs. John. Mrs. John is a 40-year-old American lady and was admitted last Friday. From her biopsy she was diagnosed with rectum cancer 6 months ago in our hospital. A colostomy was performed on her at 10:00 am yesterday. She is fully awake and recovered from the procedure. We are going to talk about her nursing implementations, especially the stoma care after the surgery.

Nurse 1：Mm, I examined her yesterday after she came back from the OR. I feel that she's doing well. Her vital signs are good, except for a slight fever. But that's normal after the surgery. The stoma is swollen, but the blood circulation around the stoma is good.

Nurse 2：Yes, we need to pay close attention to the stoma.

Head nurse：What kind of stoma is normal postoperation?

Nurse 1：Stoma is initially edematous and shrinks over the next 4 to 6 weeks. A normal stoma is moist and reddish pink. I think Mrs. John's stoma is a standard.

Head nurse：Any other signs? How about the skin?

(to be continued)

## New Words & Phrases

rectum cancer 直肠癌

biopsy n. 组织活检

colostomy n. 结肠造口术

nursing implementations 护理措施

stoma n. 造口

postoperation n. 手术后

edematous adj. 水肿的

shrink v. 收缩，退缩

### Dialogue 14　Postoperative Nursing Discussion(2)

Nurse 2：The skin is intact and free of irritation. And we should continue to monitor the condition of the stoma.

Head nurse：Good. Sounds that you know everything of the observation. Let's move on. How about the application of the pouching system? We should talk about the steps of the pouching system.

Nurse 1：The first step is to wash our hands and apply clean gloves. And then place a towel across the patient's lower abdomen to protect bed linen. Remove the used pouch and skin barrier gently.

Head nurse：Mary, do you want to follow? You must have some ideas.

Nurse 2：Mm, the skin around the stoma should be cleaned with warm water using a washcloth. Measure the stoma before cutting an opening on skin barrier. After that, the protective backing will be removed. Then apply pouch over stoma.

Head nurse：Perfect! By the way, don't forget to close the end of pouch if it is open. You guys did a wonderful job with the discussion. Thank you. Have a good day!

Nurses：You too.

## New Words & Phrases

intact adj. 完整无缺的,未经触动的,未受损伤的
irritation n. 刺激
pouching system 造瘘袋
skin barrier 皮肤黏着物
washcloth n. 擦洗布
protective backing 保护层

# Unit 8

### Dialogue 15　Enema（1）

Nurse：Hi, Mr. John. How are you today?

Patient：Not bad. How are you?

Nurse：Good. I hear you've been constipated for a few days.

Patient：Yes. I haven't had bowel movement at least 4 days so my abdomen feels distended and painful. I took some medicine but it doesn't work.

Nurse：That must be uncomfortable. Dr. Peter ordered an enema for you.

Patient：Oh, what is enema? Will it hurt?

Nurse：An enema is a tube of liquid inserted into the rectum through the anus to help your bowel movements. It won't hurt. I am sure you can handle it.

Patient：OK, I hope so. What should I do now?

Nurse：You should go to the bathroom first. I'll go to prepare the stuff and come back later.

(to be continued)

## New Words & Phrases

enema n. 灌肠剂
constipation n. 便秘
distend v. 膨胀,肿胀
rectum n. 直肠
anus n. 肛门

_Note_

stuff n. 东西

**Dialogue 16    Enema(2)**

(The nurse comes back a few minutes later)

Nurse: Mr. John. Are you ready?

Patient: Yes.

Nurse: OK, would you please show me your identification bracelet? OK, thanks. Now take off your pants to the knees and lie on your left side. Good, bend your knees, please.

Patient: Could you let me know when you start?

Nurse: Sure. Now take deep breaths. Good. Now there we go. How are you feeling now?

Patient: Is it done? I feel very uncomfortable.

Nurse: Please keep this position for 5-10 minutes and then you can go to the bathroom. Please ring the bell if you need me.

Patient: Thank you so much. I appreciate your help.

## New Words & Phrases

identification bracelet 腕带识别卡
pants n. 长裤
lie on one's left side 左侧卧位
bend the knees 屈膝
take deep breaths 深呼吸

# Unit 9

**Dialogue 17    Health Education (1)**

Nurse: Hi, Mrs. Jenny. How are you today?

Patient: Good. How are you?

Nurse: Very good. Thank you. I'd like to talk about your diabetes management before your discharge.

Patient: Oh, thanks. I am really worrying about the complications of the diabetes after I go back home.

Nurse: I understand it's not easy for you to manage it now, so we need to educate you first.

Patient: I think so.

Nurse: OK, let's start. There are two types of diabetes, type 1 and type 2. Do you know what type you have?

Patient: Type 2. It's also called the non-insulin-dependent diabetes. And the doctor suggested that I take the insulin injections.

Nurse: Good. Can you tell me how many units have been prescribed for you?

Patient: Four units of regular insulin. But I am not sure.

(to be continued)

## New Words & Phrases

diabetes n. 糖尿病

discharge n. 出院

complication n. 并发症

non-insulin-dependent diabetes 非胰岛素依赖型糖尿病

insulin n. 胰岛素

regular insulin 正规胰岛素

**Dialogue 18    Health Education（2）**

Nurse：That's correct.  Four units of insulin marks 0. 1 millimol for the 1 ml syringe.  Remember to inject the insulin 30 minutes before your meal.  It'll be more convenient for you if you can afford the insulin pen.  Most diabetics use insulin pen because its prefilled devices are disposable and easy for them.

Patient：Oh，I've heard that before.  I hope I can.

Nurse：OK.  You need to control your weight and nutrition，too.  Some regular physical activities are good for you but do not try to exercise too much at one time.  Always bring some snacks with you to prevent hypoglycemia.

Patient：OK，I see.  But it's more difficult for me to control the nutrition because I am always hungry.

Nurse：I understand.  But you must control your food according to doctors' orders in case of hyperglycemia.

Patient：My husband is always talking about that，too.  I will try.

Nurse：Good.  Here is a pocket booklet of diabetes management.  Bring it with you.

## New Words

syringe n. 注射器

diabetics n. 糖尿病患者

disposable adj. 一次性的

hypoglycemia n. 低血糖

hyperglycemia n. 高血糖

# Unit 10

**Dialogue 19    Intravenous Therapy（1）**

Nurse：Morning，Miss Susan.  I am Mary.  I will be looking after you today.

Patient：Morning，Mary.  Pleased to meet you.  How does my urine culture look?  I can't handle the pain any more.  Today I have to go to bathroom more often(今天我上卫生间的次数越来越多).

Nurse：Your urine culture indicated that you have a urinary tract infection.  And Doctor Wilson prescribed intravenous antibiotics according to your sensitivity test.

Patient：You mean you will give me an IV right now?

Nurse：Yes, if you are ready.

Patient：OK.  Do I need to take the skin test first?

Nurse：No need.  But you can go to the bathroom first and I will come back later.

Patient：Sure.  See you later.

(to be continued)

## New Words & Phrases

urine culture 尿培养
urinary tract infection 尿路感染
IV 静脉输液
sensitivity test 药敏试验
skin test 皮试

### Dialogue 20　Intravenous Therapy(2)

(A few minutes later, the nurse comes back)

Nurse：Susan, are you ready?

Patient：Yes. Will it hurt?

Nurse：Mm, just a little bit. Not much. May I check your identification bracelet first?

Patient：Sure, here you are.

Nurse：OK, thanks. Please lie down and make yourself comfortable. Hold your hand for a minute. Good. Now relax your hand. There we go.

Patient：Oh, that wasn't bad. You did a good job.

Nurse：Thank you. You'd better not to change the dripping rate. Keep your hand in whenever you move.

Patient：Alright.

Nurse：Please ring the call bell if you need help.

## New Words & Phrases

identification bracelet 腕带识别卡
dripping rate 滴速
call bell 呼叫铃

# Transcripts for Final Review

## I Listening

### Part 1

#### Extract 1

Let me examine your abdomen. Lie down on our back and bend your knees up please. It sounds like a duodenal ulcer, but we have to do some tests. Take an X-ray first, before we can be certain. You should have a complete rest and let your stomach do as little work as possible take only fluids. In addition, I'll prescribe you some medicine. If the black stools persist or your condition gets worse, come back to the hospital at once.

#### Extract 2

Mr. Gold, let me get this clear. So the pain has been basically for about two years. The X-ray is normal, but for the last two months, it's been absolutely unbearable and it's been messing up with your work and everything. I don't want to miss any detail here. Did you have an accident, a fall, or an injury? Did something, like a change, happen two months ago?

*Note*

Extract 3

I think that there's a good possibility that you have appendicitis, although one can't be sure. We'll get some blood tests checking your white blood count. However, based on your symptoms, I think that it would be wise to admit you to the hospital, and put you on a drip. If there's no improvement, I think that we should remove the appendix.

Extract 4

Hi, Jessica, your test results came in this morning. It look like you're going to need surgery to remove the tumor in your leg. After the operation, you're going to have to stay off your feet for at least three weeks. That means no soccer. The biopsy shows that the tumor is benign, which means it's not cancerous. We're going to take it out anyway just to be safe.

Extract 5

We need to remove your womb by a hysterectomy. We'll put you to sleep under a general anesthetic. We'll either make a cut in your tummy or perform the operation through the vagina. In your case, unfortunately, we'll have to remove not only the womb but also the fallopian tubes and ovaries. I'm afraid we have to do this to prevent the disease from spreading. After the operation, you won't have any periods and sadly you won't be able to have any children.

**Part 2**

The normal resting heart rate is 65-75 beats per minute. In athletes it may be as low as 40 beats per minute. In extreme athletic activity, the heart rate can go as high as 200 beats per minute. The heart rhythm may be regular or irregular. In an irregular rhythm(premature beats); or the rhythm may vary with respiration; or it may be completely irregular, as in fibrillation. When patients are aware of irregular, they describe the symptom as palpitations.

Heart failure occurs when the heart is unable to maintain sufficient cardiac output — the amount of blood pumped by the heart each minute — for the body's needs. It may involve the left side of the heart, the right side, or both. In left heart failure the main symptom is breathless. The symptom of right heart failure include peripheral oedema(swelling), beginning in the feet and ankles. This is known as pitting oedema, when a finger is pushed into swelling, it caused a small depression or pit.

**Part 3**

Interviewer: Dr. K. Vivian is an expert in the AIDS field. Today, we invite her to inform us of some basic information about HIV and AIDS. Welcome, Dr. Vivian. Because many people are quite confused about HIV and AIDS, could you please first tell us what is HIV?

Dr. K. Vivian: HIV infects cells of the immune system, destroying or impairing their functions. Infection with the virus results in progressive deterioration of the immune system, leading to "immune deficiency". The immune system is considered deficient when it can no longer fulfil its role of fighting infections and diseases.

Interviewer: And what is AIDS?

Dr. K. Vivian: AIDS is a term which applies to the most advanced stages of HIV infection. It's defined by the occurrence of any of more than 20 possible infections or HIV-related cancer.

Interviewer: Many people, including me, are quite curious about how HIV is transmitted. Could you share your ideas with us?

Dr. K. Vivian: HIV can be transmitted through unprotected sexual activities, transfusion of blood, and the sharing of dirty needles or other sharp instruments. It may also be transmitted between a mother and her infant during pregnancy, childbirth and breastfeeding.

Interviewer: How many people are living with HIV?

Dr. K. Vivian: According to estimates by the WHO, 36.9 million people were living with HIV globally at the end of 2014. That same year, some 2 million people became newly infected, and 1.2 million died of HIV-related causes.

Interviewer: How quickly does a person infected with HIV develop in AIDS?

Dr. K. Vivian: Well, the length of time can vary widely between individuals. If left without treatment, the majority of people infected with HIV will develop sighs of HIV-related illness within 5-10 years, although this can be shorter. The time between acquiring HIV and an AIDS diagnosis is usually between 10-15 years, but sometimes longer. Current treatment can slow the disease progression by preventing the virus replicating and therefore decreasing the amount of virus in an infected person's blood.

Interviewer: What's the most common life-threatening infection affecting people living with HIV/AIDS?

Dr. K. Vivian: Tuberculosis, or we usually call it TB, killed 390,000 people living with HIV in 2014. It's the number one cause of death among HIV-infected people in Africa, and a leading cause of death in this population worldwide.

Interviewer: What's the benefit of an HIV test?

Dr. K. Vivian: As far as I know, knowing your HIV status can have two important benefits. First, if you learn that you're HIV positive, you can take steps before symptoms appear to access treatment, care and support, thereby potentially prolonging your life and preventing health complications for many years. Second, if you know that you're infected, you can take measures to prevent the spread of HIV to others.

Interviewer: Is there a cure of HIV?

Dr. K. Vivian: I hate to say it, but no, there's no cure of HIV. But with good and continued treatment, the progression of HIV in the body can be slowed. Increasingly, people living with HIV can remain well and productive for extended periods of time, even in low-income countries. The WHO now recommends treatment for all people living with HIV.

Interviewer: What other kinds of care do people living with HIV need?

Dr. K. Vivian: Expect for routine treatment, people with HIV often need counseling and psychological support. Access to good nutrition, safe water and basic hygiene can also help an HIV-infected person maintain a high quality of life.

*Note*

# Appendix B  Abbreviations for Medical Use

**Part A   Abbreviations from Latin**

| | |
|---|---|
| aa | 各 |
| Abs. febr. | 不发热时 |
| Abt. ccen. | 晚饭前 |
| a. c. | 饭前 |
| ad. | 加至 |
| ad lib | 任意 |
| ad us. ext. | 外用 |
| ad us. int. | 内服 |
| Aeros. | 气雾剂 |
| a. h. | 隔 1 小时 |
| a. j. | 早饭前 |
| alt. die. | 每隔一天 |
| a. m. | 上午 |
| amp. | 安瓿 |
| a. p. | 午饭前 |
| Aq. | 水 |
| Aq. bull. | 开水 |
| Aq. cal. | 热水 |
| Aq. com. | 普通水 |
| Aq. dest. | 蒸馏水 |
| Aq. font. | 泉水 |
| Aq. gel. | 冷水 |
| Aq. steril. | 无菌水 |
| A. S. T. | 皮试后 |
| a. u. a. | 用前振摇 |
| aur. | 耳 |
| Auripil. | 耳丸剂 |
| Auristill. | 滴耳液 |
| b. i. d. | 每日两次 |
| C. | 捣碎，细切 |
| Caps. | 胶囊 |
| Catapl. | 泥剂 |
| Cit. | 迅速地 |
| Co. | 复方的 |

*Note*

| | |
|---|---|
| Collun. | 洗鼻剂 |
| Collut. | 漱口剂 |
| Collyr. | 洗眼剂 |
| Coq. | 剪、煮 |
| D. | 给予 |
| Dec. | 煎剂 |
| Degl. | 吞服 |
| Dil. | 稀释 |
| D. S. | 给予、标记 |
| D. t. d. | 给予同量 |
| Empl. | 硬膏剂 |
| Emuls. | 乳剂 |
| Enem. | 灌肠剂 |
| Extr. | 浸膏 |
| Filtr. | 过滤 |
| fl. | 花 |
| g. | 克 |
| Garg. | 含漱剂 |
| Gel. | 凝(胶)剂 |
| Gran. | 冲剂,颗粒剂 |
| Gt. | 滴,滴剂 |
| h. | 小时 |
| h. s. | 临睡前 |
| i. h. | 皮下注射 |
| i. m. | 肌内注射 |
| Inf. | 浸剂 |
| Inhal. | 吸入剂 |
| Inj. | 注射液 |
| i. v. | 静脉注射 |
| L. | 升 |
| Linim. | 擦剂 |
| Liq. | 溶液 |
| Lot. | 洗剂 |
| M. | 混合 |
| Mag. | 乳胶(剂) |
| M. D. S. | 混合给予标记 |
| M. f. m. | 混合制成合剂 |
| mg. | 毫克 |
| Mist. Mixt. | 合剂 |
| ml. | 毫升 |
| N. | 数目 |
| Nar. | 滴鼻剂 |
| Neb. | 喷雾剂 |
| Ocul. | 眼膏 |

| | |
|---|---|
| Ocus. | 眼药水 |
| O. D. | 右眼 |
| Ol. | 油剂 |
| O. S. | 左眼 |
| O. U. | 双眼 |
| Past. | 糊剂 |
| p. c. | 饭后 |
| Pell. | 膜（剂），薄膜 |
| Pil. | 丸剂 |
| p. m. | 下午 |
| p. o. | 口服 |
| pr. aur. | 耳用 |
| pr. inf. | 婴儿用 |
| pr. nar. | 鼻用 |
| p. r. n | 必要时 |
| pr. ocul | 眼用 |
| Pulv. | 粉剂，散剂 |
| q. d. | 每天 |
| q. h. | 每小时 |
| q. i. d. | 每日四次 |
| q. m. | 每天早晨 |
| q. n. | 每天晚上 |
| q. s. | 适量 |
| Rp. | 取 |
| S. | 标记 |
| Serv. | 保存 |
| s. i. d. | 每日一次 |
| Sol. | 溶液 |
| Solv. | 溶解 |
| s. o. s. | 需要时 |
| St. | 立即 |
| Supp. | 栓剂 |
| Susp. | 混悬剂 |
| Syr. | 糖浆 |
| Tab. | 片剂 |
| t. i. d. | 每日三次 |
| Tr. | 酊剂 |
| u. | 单位 |
| Ung. | 软膏 |
| ut dict. | 依医生所嘱咐 |
| vesp. | 傍晚，晚间 |

*Note*

**Part B Abbreviations from English**

| | |
|---|---|
| Ab | antibody 抗体 |
| ABG | arterial blood gas 动脉血气 |
| ACH | adrenal cortical hormone 肾上腺皮质激素 |
| ACTH | adrenocorticotropic hormone 促肾上腺皮质激素 |
| ADH | antidiuretic hormone 抗利尿激素 |
| adm | admission 入院，接收住院 |
| adm.（admin） | administration 给药 |
| ADR | adverse drug reaction 药物不良反应 |
| A/G ratio | albumin globulin ratio 白球蛋白比 |
| AI | artificial insemination 人工授精 |
| AIDS | acquired immune deficiency syndrome 获得性免疫缺陷综合征 |
| alb | albumin 白蛋白 |
| ALS | advanced life support 加强生命抢救 |
| AMI | acute myocardial infarction 急性心肌梗死 |
| ANS | autonomic nervous system 自主神经系统 |
| APTT | activated partial thromboplastin time 活化部分凝血酶时间 |
| ARDS | acute respiratory distress syndrome 急性呼吸窘迫综合征 |
| ARDS | adult respiratory distress syndrome 成人呼吸窘迫综合征 |
| ARF | acute renal failure 急性肾功能衰竭 |
| Ba | barium 钡 |
| BBT | basal body temperature 基础体温 |
| BCG | bacillus Calmette-Guerin 卡介苗 |
| BGL | blood glucose level 血糖水平 |
| bl. cult | blood culture 血培养 |
| BLS | basic life support 基础生命支持 |
| BMR | basal metabolic rate 基础代谢率 |
| BMT | bone marrow transplantation 骨髓移植 |
| BP | blood pressure 血压 |
| BPD | borderline personality disorder 边缘型人格障碍 |
| BPH | benign prostatic hyperplasia 良性前列腺增生 |
| BS | blood sugar 血糖 |
| BSL | blood sugar level 血糖水平 |
| BUN | blood urea nitrogen 血尿素氮 |
| CABG | coronary artery bypass grafting 冠状动脉旁路移植术 |
| CAD | coronary artery disease 冠状动脉疾病 |
| CA | carcinoma, cancer 肿瘤 |
| Ca | calcium 钙 |
| CAH | congenital adrenal hyperplasia 先天性肾上腺增生 |
| Cal | calorie 卡路里 |
| CAT | computed axial tomography 计算机轴向断层成像 |
| cath | catheter 导管 |
| CBC | complete blood count 全血细胞计数 |
| CC | cubic centimeter, or chief complaint 立方厘米，主诉 |

*Note*

| | |
|---|---|
| CEA | carcino-embryonic antigen 癌胚抗原 |
| CG | control group 对照组 |
| CHF | congestive heart failure 充血性心力衰竭 |
| CK | creatine kinase 肌酸激酶 |
| CKD | chronic kidney disease 慢性肾脏疾病 |
| CLL | chronic lymphocytic leukemia 慢性淋巴细胞白血病 |
| CML | chronic myelogenous leukemia 慢性髓细胞性白血病 |
| CNS | central nervous system 中枢神经系统 |
| CO | cardiac output 心输出量 |
| CO | carbon monoxide 一氧化碳 |
| $CO_2$ | carbon dioxide 二氧化碳 |
| COAD | chronic obstructive airway disease 慢性阻塞性呼吸道疾病 |
| COLD | chronic obstructive lung disease 慢性阻塞性肺疾病 |
| COPD | chronic obstructive pulmonary disease 慢性阻塞性肺疾病 |
| CPR | cardiopulmonary resuscitation 心肺复苏 |
| CRF | chronic renal failure 慢性肾功能衰竭 |
| CS | cesarean section 剖宫产 |
| CSF | cerebrospinal fluid 脑脊液 |
| CT | computed tomography 计算机断层扫描 |
| CVA | cerebrovascular accident 脑血管意外 |
| CVC | central venous catheter 中心静脉插管 |
| CVD | cardiovascular disease 脑血管疾病 |
| CVP | central venous pressure 中心静脉压 |
| CXR | chest X-ray 胸部 X 线 |
| DBP | diastolic blood pressure 舒张压 |
| DDD | daily defined doses 每日规定剂量 |
| DDx | differential diagnosis 鉴别诊断 |
| DIC | disseminated intravascular coagulation 弥散性血管内凝血 |
| DJD | degenerative joint disease 退行性关节疾病 |
| DM | diabetes mellitus 糖尿病 |
| DNA | deoxyribonucleic acid 脱氧核糖核酸 |
| DOA | dead on arrival 到达时已死 |
| DOB | date of birth 出生日期 |
| DIW | dextrose in water 葡萄糖液 |
| DU | duodenal ulcer 十二指肠溃疡 |
| ECG/EKG | electrocardiogram 心电图 |
| ED | emergency department 急诊科 |
| EDD | estimated date of delivery 预产期 |
| EDD | estimated date of discharge 预计出院日期 |
| EEG | electroencephalogram 脑电图 |
| ELISA | enzyme linked immunosorbent assay 酶联免疫吸附试验 |
| ENT | ear, nose and throat (otolaryngology) 耳鼻喉 |
| ER | emergency room 急诊室 |
| F | Fahrenheit 华氏 |

| | |
|---|---|
| FBC | full blood count 全血计数 |
| FBG | fasting blood glucose 空腹血糖 |
| FFA | free fatty acid 游离脂肪酸 |
| FHR | fetal heart rate 胎儿心率 |
| ft. | foot or feet 英尺 |
| FUO | fever of unknown origin 不明原因发热 |
| g | gram 克 |
| GA | general anaesthesia 全身麻醉 |
| gal. | gallon 加仑 |
| GH | growth hormone 生长激素 |
| GI | gastrointestinal 胃肠道的 |
| GU | gastric ulcer 胃溃疡 |
| H/A | headache 头痛 |
| HAV | hepatitis A virus 甲型肝炎病毒 |
| Hb | hemoglobin 血色素/血红蛋白 |
| HBV | hepatitis B virus 乙型肝炎病毒 |
| Hct | hematocrit 血细胞比容 |
| HCV | hepatitis C virus 丙型肝炎病毒 |
| HDL | high density lipoprotein 高密度脂蛋白 |
| HDL-C | high density lipoprotein cholesterol 高密度脂蛋白胆固醇 |
| HDV | hepatitis D virus 丁型肝炎病毒 |
| HEV | hepatitis E virus 戊型肝炎病毒 |
| HGB | hemoglobin 血色素/血红蛋白 |
| HIV | human immunodeficiency virus 人类免疫缺陷病毒 |
| HLA | human leukocyte antigen 人类白细胞抗原 |
| HR | heart rate 心率 |
| HT | hypertension 高血压 |
| IA | intraarterial 动脉内的 |
| IC | intracardiac 心脏内的 |
| ICD | International Classification of Diseases 国际疾病分类 |
| ICP | intracranial pressure 颅内压 |
| ICU | intensive care unit 重症监护病房 |
| I & D | incision and drainage 切割和引流 |
| IDA | iron deficiency anemia 缺铁性贫血 |
| IDL | intermediate density lipoprotein 中等密度脂蛋白 |
| Ig | immunoglobulin 免疫球蛋白 |
| IGT | impaired glucose tolerance 糖耐量受损 |
| i. m. | intramuscular 肌内 |
| IMI | intramuscular injection 肌内注射 |
| INF | interferon 干扰素 |
| I & O | intake and output 出入量 |
| IOP | intraocular pressure 眼内压 |
| IQ | intelligence quotient 智力商数 |
| IUCD | intrauterine contraceptive device 子宫内避孕器 |

Note

| | | |
|---|---|---|
| i. v. | intravenous 静脉内 | |
| IVDU | intravenous drug user 静脉注射吸毒者 | |
| IVP | intravenous pyelogram 静脉注射肾盂造影 | |
| kg | kilogram 千克 | |
| LDH | lactate dehydrogenase 乳酸盐脱氢酶 | |
| LDL | low density lipoprotein 低密度脂蛋白 | |
| LDL-C | low density lipoprotein cholesterol 低密度脂蛋白胆固醇 | |
| Leu | leukocytes 白细胞 | |
| LFT | liver function test 肝功能测试 | |
| LMP | last menstrual period 末次月经 | |
| Lp | lipoprotein 脂蛋白 | |
| LP | lumbar puncture 腰椎穿刺 | |
| LPL | lipoprotein lipase 脂蛋白脂肪酶 | |
| LUL | left upper lobe 左上叶 | |
| Ly | lymphocyte 淋巴细胞 | |
| MAP | mean artery pressure 平均动脉压 | |
| MCD | mean corpuscular diameter 红细胞平均直径 | |
| MCH | mean cell hemoglobin 红细胞平均血红蛋白 | |
| MCHC | mean cell hemoglobin concentration 红细胞平均血红蛋白浓度 | |
| MCV | mean cell volume 细胞平均容积 | |
| Mg | magnesium 镁 | |
| MI | myocardial infarction 心肌梗死 | |
| Mod | moderate 中等的 | |
| Mo | monocyte 单核细胞 | |
| MPV | mean platelet volume 血小板平均容积 | |
| MRA | magnetic resonance angiogram or angiography 磁共振血管造影 | |
| MRI | magnetic resonance imaging 磁共振成像 | |
| NA | nursing assistant 护理员 | |
| NAD | no abnormality detected 未见异常 | |
| NBM | nothing by mouth 禁食 | |
| NE | norepinephrine 去甲肾上腺素 | |
| Neo | neoplasm 肿瘤 | |
| NIDDM | non-insulin-dependent diabetes mellitus Ⅱ型糖尿病 | |
| Npl | neoplasm 肿瘤 | |
| NREM | non-rapid eye movement 非快速眼动 | |
| NS | normal saline 生理盐水 | |
| NTG | nitroglycerin 硝化甘油 | |
| N&V | nausea & vomiting 恶心和呕吐 | |
| NVD | nausea, vomiting & diarrhea 恶心、呕吐和腹泻 | |
| NVD | normal vaginal delivery 正常阴道分娩 | |
| $O_2$ | oxygen 氧 | |
| OA | osteoarthritis 骨关节炎 | |
| OB-GYN | obstetrics and gynecology 产科与妇科 | |
| OD | overdose 剂量过多 | |

| OGTT | oral glucose tolerance test 口服葡萄糖耐量试验 |
|---|---|
| OP | outpatient department 门诊部 |
| OS | orthopedic surgery 整形外科 |
| OR | operating room 手术室 |
| OTC | over-the-counter drug 非处方药 |
| PA | pulmonary artery 肺动脉 |
| PAH | pulmonary arterial hypertension 肺动脉高压 |
| PE | pulmonary embolism 肺栓塞 |
| PE | physical examination 体格检查 |
| PLT | platelet 血小板 |
| Post-op | postoperative 手术后的 |
| PPH | post partum hemorrhage 产后出血 |
| PPH | primary pulmonary hypertension 原发性肺动脉高压 |
| Pre-op | preoperative 手术前的 |
| PT | physical therapy 物理治疗 |
| PVD | peripheral vascular disease 外周血管疾病 |
| PVR | pulmonary vascular resistance 肺血管阻力 |
| Px | physical examination 体格检查 |
| Prog | prognosis 预后 |
| RA | refractory anaemia 难治性贫血 |
| RA | rheumatoid arthritis 风湿性关节炎 |
| RAI | radioactive iodine 放射性碘 |
| RBC | red blood cell count 红细胞计数 |
| REM | rapid eye movement 快速眼动 |
| RF | rheumatoid factor 类风湿因子 |
| RFT | renal function test 肾脏功能测试 |
| RhF | rheumatoid factor 类风湿因子 |
| RLQ | right lower quadrant 右下腹部 |
| ROM | range of motion 环绕关节运动,全关节运动图 |
| RR | respiratory rate 呼吸频率 |
| RT | radiotherapy 放射治疗 |
| RUQ | right upper quadrant 右上腹部 |
| RV | right ventricle 右心室 |
| RVF | right ventricular failure 右心室衰竭 |
| RVSP | right ventricular systolic pressure 右心室收缩压 |
| SARS | severe acute respiratory syndrome 严重急性呼吸道综合征 |
| SBE | subacute bacterial endocarditis 亚急性感染性心内膜炎 |
| SBP | systolic blood pressure 收缩压 |
| SBP | spontaneous bacterial peritonitis 自发性细菌腹膜炎 |
| SHx | surgical history 手术史 |
| SLE | systemic lupus erythematosus 系统性红斑狼疮 |
| SOB | shortness of breath 气促 |
| SOS | save our souls, meaning "in case of emergency" 急救 |
| ST | skin test 皮试 |

Note

| STD | sexually transmitted disease 性传播疾病 |
| STI | soft tissue injury 软组织损伤 |
| Subq | subcutaneous 皮下 |
| SVI | systemic viral infection 系统性病毒感染 |
| Syr | syrup 糖浆 |
| TB | tuberculosis 肺结核 |
| TF | transfer 转院,转科 |
| T/F | transfer 转院,转科 |
| THR | total hip replacement 全髋关节置换术 |
| TIA | transient ischemic attack 短暂性脑缺血发作 |
| TKR | total knee replacement 全膝关节置换术 |
| TLC | total lung capacity 肺总容量 |
| TOP | termination of pregnancy 妊娠终止 |
| TPN | total parenteral nutrition 全胃肠道外营养 |
| TSH | thyroid stimulating hormone 促甲状腺激素 |
| TT | thrombin time 凝血酶时间 |
| TTE | transthoracic echocardiogram 经胸廓心回波图 |
| Tu | tumor 肿瘤 |
| TUR | transurethral resection 经尿道切除术 |
| Tx | transplant 移植 |
| UBT | urea breath test 尿素呼气试验 |
| URTI | upper respiratory tract infection 上呼吸道感染 |
| US | ultrasound 超声 |
| USG | ultrasonography 超声波检查法 |
| USS | ultrasound scan 超声波扫描 |
| UTI | urinary tract infection 尿路感染 |
| VA | visual acuity 视觉敏度 |
| VC | vital capacity 肺活量 |
| VD | vaginal delivery 产道分娩 |
| VE | vaginal examination (manual examination)阴道检查 |
| VF | ventricular fibrillation 心室颤动 |
| VLDL | very low density lipoprotein 极低密度脂蛋白 |
| WBC | white blood cell count 白细胞计数 |

# Appendix C　Text Translation

## Unit 1　The Cardiovascular System

课文 A

### 中国的心血管系统疾病现状

**心脏和循环系统**

心脏和循环系统(也称为心血管系统)构成向机体组织输送血液的网络。随着每次心跳,血液被输送到全身,把氧和营养物质带到人体所有细胞。

每天,体内约有 10 品脱(5 L)血液在大约 6 万英里(96560 km)的血管里反复循环,这些血管分出分支并相互交联形成通路,连接人体器官和身体各部位的细胞。从一直搏动的心脏,到厚壁的大动脉,直到通过显微镜才能看到的细小的毛细血管网,心血管系统构成了人体的生命线。

循环系统由心脏和血管组成,后者包括动脉、静脉和毛细血管。实际上人体有两个循环系统:肺循环是一个较短的回路,从心脏到双肺往返不止,体循环(也就是人们经常认为的人体循环系统)把血液从心脏送到身体其他各个部位并循环往复。

**我国的心血管系统疾病**

我国心血管系统疾病发病率的增高似乎在很大程度上由高血压的增多引起。体质指数(BMI)上升、体育锻炼减少、吸烟人群的比例居高不下、不健康饮食也都导致越来越重的心血管系统疾病负担,心血管系统疾病居我国死亡原因首位。

广泛的饮食、生活方式和代谢等风险因素可能一直在影响我国的心血管系统疾病负担。我国社会的急剧变化,包括从传统到更"西式"的饮食和生活习惯、快速的城市化和工业化,导致诸如心脏病和脑卒中等心血管系统疾病的增加。在我国人群中,这些变化伴随着高胆固醇、肥胖和 Ⅱ 型糖尿病的显著增多。通过促进健康饮食和生活方式预防心血管系统疾病应上升为国家优先公共政策。

课文 B

### 高血压

全世界约有 10 亿人患有高血压,它是人类发病和死亡的主要原因之一。许多人没有意识到他们已患有高血压。因此,这种疾病有时被称为"沉默的杀手"。这种疾病通常是无症状的,直至观察到高血压的靶器官损害症状(如脑卒中、心肌梗死、肾功能不全、视力问题等)。

高血压被定义为血压的异常升高。收缩压和舒张压数值都应被重视。根据美国的一些高血压诊断指南,可用下表数值描述高血压的不同阶段。

| 分　类 | 收缩压/mmHg | 舒张压/mmHg |
|---|---|---|
| 正常 | <120 | <80 |
| 临界 | 120～139 | 80～89 |

续表

| 分　类 | 收缩压/mmHg | 舒张压/mmHg |
|---|---|---|
| 第一阶段 | 140～160 | 90～100 |
| 第二阶段 | ＞160 | ＞100 |

对于 90％～95％ 的高血压患者,病因尚不清楚,这种情况称为原发性高血压。其余 5％～10％ 的高血压患者是由于肾病、内分泌疾病,或其他可明确病因而继发的,这种高血压称为继发性高血压。

高血压危象指可能导致脑卒中的血压急剧升高。血压急剧升高(超过 180/110 mmHg)将损害血管。心脏可能不能维持足够的血液循环。高血压危象分为高血压急症和高血压危症两类。高血压急症的体征和症状包括血压升高,严重头痛,严重焦虑和呼吸短促。高血压危症患者会出现肺水肿、脑水肿或脑出血、心脏病发作、脑卒中等威胁生命的体征和症状。

医生不能确定大多数高血压患者的病因。但现已公认有几种情况会导致血压升高,如肥胖、酗酒、有高血压家族史、盐摄入过多、衰老等。体力锻炼减少、钾和钙摄取不足也可能使血压升高。

高血压一般不会产生症状。大多数患者因其他原因就医时才被告知他们患有高血压。如果不经治疗,高血压会损害心脏、大脑、肾或眼睛。其损害会导致冠心病、脑卒中和肾功能衰竭等问题。非常高的血压会导致头痛、视力问题、恶心和呕吐。

高血压的治疗取决于患者具体血压值的高低,是否合并有糖尿病等其他健康问题,以及是否有其他脏器功能损害。医生也会考虑患者患上其他疾病,特别是心脏病的可能性。大多数高血压患者服用降压药物治疗。高血压也常用降低心输出量的药物来治疗。血管舒张类药物可降低全身血管阻力,也可用于治疗高血压。

人们可以通过采用健康的生活方式来降低血压。如果这些生活方式的改变不起作用,则可能需要服用药物。有助于预防高血压的生活方式的改变如下。

· 减肥。

· 减少盐的摄入量。

· 锻炼。

· 限制酒精摄入量。

· 每日饮食摄入 3500 mg 钾。新鲜的、未加工的食物钾含量最高,如肉、鱼、无脂或低脂奶制品、多种水果和蔬菜。

## Unit 2　The Digestive System

课文 A

### 消化系统简介

我们所吃的所有食物都必须被分解成可以被身体吸收的营养物质,这就是为什么需要数小时才能充分消化食物。在人体中,蛋白质必须分解成氨基酸,淀粉分解成单糖,脂肪分解成脂肪酸和甘油。食物和饮料中的水也会被吸收到血液中,为身体提供所需的液体。

消化系统由消化道和其他参与消化的腹部器官组成,如肝脏和胰腺。消化道是从口腔到肛门的一个长管,包括食管、胃和肠等器官。成年人的消化道大约有 30 英尺(9.144 m)长。

消化过程在食物到达胃之前就开始了。当我们看到、闻到、尝到,甚至想象美味的小吃时,位于我们舌头下和下颌附近的唾液腺就开始分泌唾液。这种唾液的流动是由大脑反射引起的,当我们感觉到食物,甚至想吃东西时,大脑反射就会触发。作为对这种感觉刺激的反应,大脑通过控制唾液腺的神经发出准备吃饭的信号。

在吸收过程中,来自食物的营养物质(包括碳水化合物、蛋白质、脂肪、维生素和矿物质)通过肠壁的通道进入血液。血液将这些营养物质分配给身体的其他部分。身体不能使用的食物的废弃部分作为粪便排出体外。

**课文 B**

### 便秘

便秘是消化系统中常见的健康问题之一,其表现为排便次数减少,粪便干结,或者排便困难,有时甚至好几天都不排便。

即使不是天天排便,也不能就此下结论说是便秘。判断是便秘的话,还应有以下表现:粪便干结且一周内排便次数少于 3 次;排便困难经常发作;腹胀或其他腹部不适。

要进一步理解什么是便秘,就要了解结肠或者大肠是怎样运转的。当食物残渣随着肠蠕动进入大肠后,其中一部分水分被大肠吸收,形成粪便。粪便随着肠蠕动到达直肠,之后变成固体,因为大部分的水分被吸收。

若大肠吸收的水分过多或者肠蠕动减慢使粪便在肠道中停留时间过长,就会导致便秘。结果使大便变得干燥坚硬。通常情况下,引起便秘的因素如下。

- 水分摄入不足。
- 食物中缺少纤维。
- 没有养成良好的排便习惯。
- 年龄。
- 缺乏运动。
- 怀孕。
- 疾病。

当发生便秘时,你会感到排便比平时困难。因为一个或者更多的原因,排便变得更加困难。比如,排便的次数减少,无效排便(感觉排便不尽)。

大多数患有便秘的人不必过分担心,只有少数便秘的人存在严重的医学问题。如果你已经有两个星期以上没有排便,那就要去医院就诊,以确诊病因并及时治疗。如果便秘是由结肠癌引起的,早诊断、早治疗就显得非常重要。

便秘的诊断通常依赖于病史和物理检查。医生首先会想办法确定小肠或者直肠有没有阻塞(肠梗阻),然后确定激素水平是否正常,比如是否存在甲状腺功能减退或者电解质失衡。医生还会了解你的药物使用情况,这些药物可能是引发你便秘的原因。

如果便秘不是由医学问题引起的,就可以通过饮食来调节,比如多喝水,多吃一些纤维素含量丰富的食物(纤维素可以从大量的蔬菜、水果、面食中获得)以及增加饮食中亚麻油的含量。这些常规的非处方通便方法被人们忽视,原因可能是这些通便方法导致肠蠕动变得有依赖性。灌肠可作为一种医学治疗方法来解除便秘。然而,灌肠通常只用于由直肠原因引起的便秘,而非作用于整个肠道系统。

# Unit 3   The Respiratory System

**课文 A**

### 普通感冒

普通感冒,亦称上呼吸道感染,是一种由诸多不同类型病毒所致的传染性疾病。由于导致感冒的病毒数量众多,以及新的病毒不断出现,人体不能对所有感冒相关病毒都产生抵抗力,因此,感冒易频发和复发。

普通感冒的症状有鼻塞、流鼻涕、咽喉疼痛、声音嘶哑、咳嗽,还有可能包括发热和头痛。许多感冒患者感到疲倦和疼痛。这些症状一般会持续 3～10 天。

无论患者是否服药，感冒经常会在几天到数周内好转。但是，病毒会引起其他感染侵袭人体，这些感染包括鼻窦感染、耳部感染和支气管炎。即使在感冒消失后，哮喘、慢性支气管炎或肺气肿患者的症状也可能在数周内加重。

普通感冒大多通过手部接触传染。例如，感冒患者流鼻涕，用手接触鼻子，然后接触其他人，其他人就会被病毒感染。此外，人们还可能被钢笔、书籍、咖啡杯子等物体上的病毒感染。尽管常识表明咳嗽和打喷嚏会传播病毒，但事实上这些并非传播病毒的常见方式。

一般来说，抗生素治疗对感冒并无疗效。抗生素只是对细菌导致的疾病有疗效，而感冒通常由病毒所致。抗生素不仅没有帮助，反而可能导致致命的过敏反应。还有，滥用抗生素已经导致几种常见细菌对抗生素产生了耐药性。由于上述及其他原因，限制抗生素的使用显得十分重要。有时，病毒引发感冒后会出现细菌感染，普通感冒产生的细菌性并发症可用抗生素治疗。

有几种缓解感冒症状的疗法。解充血药和鼻用喷剂有助于缓解感冒症状。心脏病患者、高血压控制不良者和患有其他疾病者在使用这些药物之前应该与医生联系。而且，鼻用喷剂非处方药的使用不应超过 3 天，因为鼻部可能产生依赖性，中止使用这些药物可能会产生更严重的鼻塞。

**课文 B**

### 禽流感

禽流感也称 H5N1。这种疾病与猪流感、犬流感、马流感和人类流感相似，都是由已适应某特定物种的不同株系流感病毒所致。

禽类像人类一样会患上流感。禽流感病毒感染对象包括鸡、鸭、其他家禽和野生鸟类等禽类。然而，禽流感会对人类的健康产生威胁。1997 年在中国香港出现了第一例直接感染人类的禽流感病毒 H5N1。此后，禽流感病毒扩散到亚洲、非洲和欧洲的许多国家。

人类感染禽流感病毒虽然少见，但是导致鸟类感染的病毒会变化或变异，然后更容易使人类感染。这样会导致禽流感大范围流行，或在全世界暴发。

在禽流感病毒暴发期间，与感染禽类接触过的人群会患病。吃没有煮熟的家禽或接触已感染人群也可能使人患病。禽流感病毒会使人重病甚至会致人死亡。目前还没有出现能预防该疾病的疫苗。

禽流感病毒在鸟类中自然存在。全世界的野生鸟类的肠道中存在这种病毒，但它们一般不会因此患病。然而，禽流感病毒在家禽中传染性很强，会使鸡、鸭、火鸡等家禽患病身亡。

感染了禽流感病毒的鸟类的唾液、鼻涕和粪便中包含病毒。易感鸟类在接触此类含病毒的分泌物或排泄物时，或接触被此类分泌物或排泄物污染的物体表面时，就会感染禽流感病毒。家禽感染禽流感病毒的途径有直接接触已感染水禽或家禽，或接触被禽流感病毒污染的表面（如尘土或鸟笼）或物质（如水或饲料）。

人类禽流感的症状有典型的流感样症状（如发热、咳嗽、咽喉肿痛和肌肉疼痛）、眼睛感染、肺炎、严重呼吸道疾病（例如急性呼吸道窘迫），以及其他严重威胁生命的并发症。禽流感的症状取决于导致感染的病毒类型。

已有实验室研究表明一些处方药在治疗人类禽流感病毒感染方面应该有效。但是，禽流感病毒会对这些药物产生耐药性，因此这些药物并非总是有效。人们需要更多的研究来证实这些药物的有效性。

# Unit 4　The Nervous System

**课文 A**

### 大脑和神经系统介绍

**大脑和神经系统在日常生活中的作用**

如果将大脑比作一台中央电脑，控制着身体的所有功能，那么神经系统就像一个网络，将信息从大脑传送到身体的不同部位。它通过脊髓完成这一过程，脊髓从大脑向下延伸到背部，内含有细细的管束状的神经,延伸到身体的每个器官和组织。

当信息从身体的任何部位进入大脑时,大脑会告诉身体如何做出反应。例如,如果你不小心碰到了一个热火炉,你的皮肤中的神经就会向你的大脑发出疼痛的信号。然后大脑马上传回一条信息,告诉手上的肌肉赶紧将手拿开。幸运的是,这种神经传递花费的时间比你阅读这段话花费的时间要少得多!

### 大脑如何运行

大脑重约 3 磅,考虑到它所做的一切工作,人类的大脑真是令人难以置信的紧凑。它的许多褶皱和凹槽为它提供了储存身体所有重要信息所必需的额外表面积。

脊髓是一长束神经组织,长约 18 英寸、厚 3/4 英寸。它从大脑底部向下延伸至脊柱。在这一过程中,各种神经分支到全身。这些构成了外周神经系统。

大脑和脊髓都被骨骼保护。大脑由颅骨保护,脊髓由组成脊柱的一套环形骨骼即被称为椎骨的骨骼保护。它们都被多层膜和一种特殊的体液缓冲保护,前者称为脑膜,后者称为脑脊液。这些体液有助于保护神经组织,让它保持健康状态,并清除废物。

### 课文 B

#### 脑 PET 扫描

脑部正电子发射断层成像(PET)是脑部的一种成像检查。它使用一种被称为示踪剂的放射性物质来寻找脑部的疾病和损伤。这种扫描可以显示大脑及其组织如何运作。其他的成像检查,如磁共振成像(MRI)和计算机断层扫描(CT)仅能显示脑部的结构。

正电子发射断层成像(PET)扫描需要少量放射性物质(示踪剂),这种示踪剂通常通过肘部附近的静脉注入。示踪剂流经人体血液后在器官和组织中停留,它可以帮助医生(通常是放射科医生)更加清楚地看到某些部位或某些疾病。

患者躺在一张狭窄的桌板上,然后滑入一个大型隧道型扫描仪。正电子发射断层成像扫描仪会检测器官和组织中的示踪剂,计算机将这些结果转换成 3D 图像。图像会显示在监测器上,供医生或护士阅览。

这种检查有以下用途。

• 诊断癌症和恶性肿瘤。

• 为癫痫手术做准备。

• 帮助诊断阿尔茨海默病。

• 鉴别帕金森病和其他运动障碍疾病。

医生可以通过几次正电子发射断层成像(PET)扫描来确定患者对癌症或其他疾病的治疗反应情况。这种检查花费的时间在 30 min 到 2 h 之间。

## Unit 5　The Endocrine and Lymphatic Systems

### 课文 A

#### 内分泌与淋巴系统

##### 什么是内分泌系统?

虽然我们很少会想到内分泌系统,但它几乎影响我们身体的每一个细胞、器官和功能。内分泌系统在调节情绪、生长发育、组织功能、新陈代谢、性功能和生殖过程等方面发挥着重要作用。

一般来说,内分泌系统负责身体一些缓慢发生的过程,如细胞生长。呼吸和身体运动等较快的过程是由神经系统控制的。尽管神经系统和内分泌系统是相互独立的系统,但它们经常协同工作以帮助身体正常运作。

内分泌系统的基础是激素和腺体。作为身体的化学信使,激素将信息和指令从一组细胞传递到另

145

一组细胞。不同的激素随着血流在体内流动,但每种激素只会影响某些特定的细胞。腺体是一组产生、分泌或释放化学物质的细胞。腺体选择和移除血液中的物质,对其进行加工,然后分泌出最终的化学物质,以供身体所需。

**什么是淋巴系统?**

淋巴系统是一个广泛的引流网络,有助于保持体液平衡,保护身体免受感染。淋巴系统是由淋巴管网络组成的。这些淋巴管内流淌的淋巴液(一种透明的含有蛋白质、盐、葡萄糖、尿素和其他物质的液体)遍布全身。脾脏位于胸腔下腹部的左上部分。它作为淋巴系统的一个部分来保护身体,清除血液中衰亡的红细胞和其他异物,帮助抵御感染。

**课文 B**

### 中国糖尿病情况及预防建议

中国过去几十年的经济增长极大地改变了国家的经济格局,使 5 亿人摆脱了贫困。然而,伴随这一进展而来的是一些疾病的增加,如糖尿病,这主要与城市化发展和生活方式的改变有关。25 年前,中国患有糖尿病的人数占比不到 1%。如今,中国有超过 1.14 亿人患有糖尿病,是世界上患糖尿病人数最多的国家。

据估计,中国成年人中有 11.6% 患有糖尿病,高于美国的 11.3%。专家将此归咎于久坐不动的生活方式、高糖高热量的西方化饮食、过度吸烟和缺乏锻炼。一些专家表示,2007 年至 2025 年间,印度和中国的糖尿病患者人数将增加 4850 万。

糖尿病分为两种,1 型糖尿病主要在儿童和年轻人中确诊,可能有遗传和环境因素的影响。2 型糖尿病可能也有小部分遗传的因素,主要还是由不健康的生活方式和肥胖引起的。1 型糖尿病约占所有病例的 5%。

2 型糖尿病是最常见的一种糖尿病,预防是非常重要的。如果你患糖尿病的风险较高,比如超重或者有家族病史,那么预防糖尿病就尤为重要。

**1. 多做体育活动**

有规律的体育活动有很多好处。运动可以帮助你减肥,降低血糖和提升对胰岛素的敏感性,有助于保持你的血糖在正常范围内。

研究表明有氧运动和阻力训练可以帮助控制糖尿病。两者结合的运动计划能取得最佳效果。

**2. 摄入大量纤维**

纤维的口感粗糙,并不可口,但它能帮助你通过改善血糖控制减少患糖尿病的危险,降低患心脏病的风险,增加饱腹感以利于减肥。

高纤维食物包括水果、蔬菜、豆类、全谷物和坚果。

**3. 吃全谷类食品**

尽管目前还不清楚原因,但全谷类食品可以降低患糖尿病的风险,帮助维持血糖水平。尽量让你的谷物中至少有一半是全谷物。许多由全谷物制成的食物可以随时食用,包括各种面包、面食和麦片。在包装和成分表的前几项中寻找"全谷"这个词。

**4. 减重**

如果你超重,预防糖尿病可能取决于减肥。你减掉的每一磅体重都能改善你的健康状况,你可能会惊讶于它的改善程度。在一项大型研究中,适度减轻体重(减少约初始体重的 7%)并定期锻炼的参与者,患糖尿病的风险降低了近 60%。

**5. 丢弃网红饮食法,做出更健康的选择**

低碳水饮食法、血糖指数饮食法或其他网红饮食法可能会帮助你在初始阶段减肥。但它们预防糖尿病的效果尚不明确,长期效果也不清楚。如果你不吃或严格限制摄入某种食物,你可能就丢失了必需的营养。相反,健康饮食中应该具有多样性和分量控制。

# Unit 6　The Immune System

## 课文 A

### 应对中国罕见的遗传病

中国拥有 14 亿人口,是世界上罕见遗传病患者人数最多的国家。据目前估计,患有染色体疾病的人数超过 1000 万,患有单基因疾病的人数也超过 100 万。

遗传病可分为染色体疾病和单基因疾病,全球大约有 1% 的人口发病。迄今,已发现 100 多种不同的染色体疾病。染色体疾病被认为是在人类发展早期出现的。最常见的染色体疾病是唐氏综合征(DS),每 700 个新生儿中就有 1 个唐氏综合征患儿。

由于缺乏可用的和可负担的治疗方法,罕见遗传病患者的护理需求在很大程度上无法得到满足。因此,近年来,公众越来越认识到政府、医疗单位、临床医生和患者都需要采取积极行动来满足上述需求。

全基因组测序等新一代测序技术(NGS)的出现,为在中国人群中进行大规模的人口筛查,确定罕见遗传病的分子病因提供了新的机遇。因缺乏有效治疗手段,中国近期研究并实施的一种替代手段——无创 DNA 产前检测(NIPT),是最有可能减少出生时患有罕见遗传病儿童数量的单一技术。

尽管中国的遗传病患者数量非常大,但大多数患者待在家里,不参与日常社交活动。除了为相关疾病或残疾人群举行的特别活动外,遗传病患者很少出现在公共场合。和许多其他文化一样,中国的传统价值观不鼓励家中的患者外出。由于不了解疾病的原因,过去社会往往把残疾归咎于家庭。此外,在家庭内部,当一个孩子出生时就带有遗传病,父母中有一方很有可能会强烈地指责另一方损害了家庭声誉,让家人蒙羞。

在中国,家庭应对遗传病的方式正在发生着文化观念的转变。现在,越来越多的家庭和患者选择就医,通过寻求医生关于疾病的医学建议和可能的治疗方法来减轻痛苦。医生在对大多数遗传病做出正确的临床诊断方面越来越熟练,一些患者愿意支付少量的 DNA 检测费用,以确定家族突变的基因。如果家庭成员已经结婚并有生育计划,产前诊断将成为一个重要的步骤。

一旦父母对孩子的疾病和可能的治疗方法有了更好的了解,他们就更容易接受疾病,能更从容地应对疾病负担给家庭带来的长期影响。

## 课文 B

### 艾滋病

20 多年来,人们一直被警告要提防艾滋病病毒和艾滋病。艾滋病已经夺去了数百万人的生命,是当今世界面临的极大问题之一,没有人能摆脱它的影响。每个人都应该了解艾滋病的基本情况。AIDS 是获得性免疫缺陷综合征的缩写。它是由于感染了一种被称为 HIV 的病毒,即人类免疫缺陷病毒。这种疾病主要通过性行为和血液传播。这种病毒攻击人体中一种称为 CD4 阳性($CD4^+$)T 细胞的关键细胞,这些细胞是人体免疫系统非常重要的部分,可以对抗感染和各种癌症。

**2007 年关于世界艾滋病和 HIV 流行的最新统计数字**

| | | |
|---|---|---|
| HIV<br>感染者/艾滋病患者 | 总数 | 33,200,000 (30,600,000~36,100,000) |
| | 成人 | 30,800,000 (28,200,000~33,600,000) |
| | 女性 | 15,400,000 ( 13,900,000~16,600,000) |
| | 15 岁及以下儿童 | 2,500,000 (2,200,000~2,600,000) |

*Note*

| HIV<br>新发感染者/艾滋病患者 | 总数 | 2,500,000 (1,800,000~4,100,000) |
|---|---|---|
| | 成人 | 2,100,000 (1,400,000~3,600,000) |
| | 15岁及以下儿童 | 420,000(350,000~540,000) |
| 感染 HIV 死亡人数 | 总数 | 2,100,000 (1,900,000~2,400,000) |
| | 成人 | 1,700,000 (1,600,000~2,100,000) |
| | 15岁及以下儿童 | 330,000 (310,000~380,000) |

由于发生机会性感染的内脏器官和肿瘤发生的部位不同,艾滋病症状复杂多样。

常见症状如下:

·一般症状:持续发热、虚弱、盗汗、全身浅表淋巴结肿大、消瘦。

·呼吸系统症状:长期咳嗽、胸痛、呼吸困难、严重时痰中带血。

·消化道症状:厌食、恶心、呕吐、腹泻、严重时便血。

·神经系统症状:头晕、头痛、反应迟钝、智力减退、精神异常、抽搐、偏瘫、痴呆。

·皮肤和黏膜症状:单纯疱疹、带状疱疹、口腔和咽部黏膜炎症及溃烂。

此外,可出现多种恶性肿瘤,如位于体表的卡波西肉瘤,可见红色或紫红色的斑疹、丘疹和浸润性肿块。

由此可见,艾滋病的症状非常复杂。

HIV 感染可以通过检测血液中存在的 HIV 抗体(一种抗病毒蛋白)来明确诊断。可以采用两种不同类型的抗体试验,即酶联免疫吸附试验(ELISA)和免疫印迹检测。

你可以通过避免高危行为来减少感染 HIV 的机会:

·杜绝不洁性行为,对伴侣保持忠诚。

·正确使用安全套。

·如需静脉注射,不要与他人共用注射器。

·如果你是医疗卫生工作者,严格执行通用预防措施(避免体液接触的感染防控程序)

·如果你是一名想要怀孕的女性,事先要做 HIV 检测,特别是如果你有感染 HIV 风险的行为史。HIV 呈阳性的孕妇需要特殊的产前护理和药物,以减少将 HIV 传染给新生儿的风险。

自 20 世纪 90 年代中期以来,人们对艾滋病的预防和治疗有了显著的改善,但迄今仍然没有办法治愈艾滋病。治疗的一般原则是抗感染、抗肿瘤、消除或抑制 HIV、改善机体免疫功能。

## Unit 7   The Urinary System

课文 A

### 尿路感染

才上午 10 点,那天早上特蕾西已经去了 6 次厕所。有时她几乎没有时间征求老师同意,因为她小便很急。是她早餐喝了太多橙汁吗? 没有——虽然她不得不去洗手间,但每次的尿液都很少。每次小便的时候,她都有一种灼热感。这到底是什么情况?

特蕾西的这种经历并不少见。她的问题是尿路感染,这是青少年尤其是女孩生病看医生常见的原因之一。

细菌性尿路感染(UTI)是影响泌尿道最常见的一种感染。尿,或称尿液,是由肾脏从血液中过滤出来的液体。尿液含有盐和代谢产物,通常不含细菌。当细菌进入膀胱或肾脏并在尿液中繁殖时,就会导致 UTI。

UTI 主要有三种类型。细菌仅感染尿道(将尿液从膀胱输送到体外的短管)会引起尿道炎。

细菌也能引起膀胱感染,称为膀胱炎。另一种更严重的尿路感染是肾脏本身感染,称为肾盂肾炎。患有这种尿路感染的患者,通常会伴有背部疼痛、高烧和呕吐。

最常见的尿路感染是膀胱感染,大多只是造成不适和不便。膀胱感染可以迅速且较容易地治疗。为避免更严重的肾脏感染,及时接受治疗非常重要。请记住,尽管尿路感染让人很不适,而且往往很痛苦,但这非常常见,也很容易治疗。只要及时就医就能尽早摆脱这个问题。

**课文 B**

### 急性肾功能衰竭

急性肾功能衰竭是指肾脏排泄功能(即从血液中滤过多余液体和代谢产物的功能)在短时间内急剧下降,引起水、电解质紊乱及代谢产物蓄积。

急性肾功能衰竭最常见于住院患者,尤其是重症监护患者。急性肾功能衰竭常继发于复杂手术,严重损伤,或肾缺血患者。

肾功能可随着时间或疾病进展逐渐下降,在疾病早期,临床表现或症状不明显。这种情况通常被称为慢性肾功能衰竭,高血压和糖尿病是引起慢性肾功能衰竭常见的原因。

急性肾功能衰竭可出现严重情况,通常需要强化治疗。然而,与慢性肾功能衰竭不同,急性肾功能衰竭是可逆的,如果你身体状况良好,肾功能在几周内即可恢复正常。如果急性肾功能衰竭发生在严重慢性疾病的病程中,如心脏病发作、脑卒中、重症感染,结果往往更糟。

急性肾功能衰竭的临床表现和症状包括以下几种。

· 尿量减少,虽然偶尔排尿正常。

· 液体潴留,导致腿、踝部或足部水肿。

· 嗜睡。

· 呼吸短促。

· 疲劳。

· 代谢紊乱。

· 重症患者可出现癫痫或昏迷。

· 由心包炎(覆盖在心脏表面的囊状膜的炎性反应)引起的胸痛等。

部分患者没有注意到早期临床表现或症状,但因导致突发肾功能衰竭的潜在问题而焦虑。

肾脏是两个蚕豆状的器官,每个约拳头大小,位于脊柱两侧,紧贴腹后壁,居腹膜后方。肾脏滤过血液中的多余液体,排出代谢产物。血液首先通过主动脉(将血液从心脏输送到全身的主要动脉)的分支——肾动脉进入肾,然后从肾动脉流向每个肾单位。

每个肾脏包含约 100 万个肾单位,每个肾单位由一簇毛细血管(肾小球)和肾小管组成,肾小管通向更大的集合管。人体的血液均从肾小球滤过。

滤过后的物质进入肾小管,包括代谢产物和人体健康所需的重要物质。尿素、尿酸和肌酐等代谢产物在肾脏通过尿液排出,而身体所需物质,如糖、氨基酸、钙和盐,则被重吸收回血液中。

# Unit 8　The Musculoskeletal System

**课文 A**

### 儿童骨折的增加

在全国范围内,医生报告骨折儿童的数量稳步上升。

华盛顿哥伦比亚特区的儿科整形外科医生劳拉托西说:"目前的事实是,儿童身体各部位都可骨折。肘部骨折的发病率非常高,手臂中部和手部的骨折也是如此。"梅奥诊所最近发表的一项研究发现在过去 30 年里,该市男孩的前臂骨折增加了 32% 以上,女孩增加了 56%。研究人员表示,他们不确定骨折发病率上升的原因。但他们怀疑一个主要原因是儿童摄入钙不足,而钙是强健骨骼的必要元素。

"当今美国儿童的饮食中主要缺乏钙。"杜安·亚历山大医生说。根据美国农业部的统计数据,86%的青春期女孩和 64% 的青春期男孩"缺钙";换言之,他们没有摄入推荐的每日钙摄入量(RDA),即 1300 毫克,相当于每天 4 杯 8 盎司的牛奶。

亚历山大说:"在过去的 20 年到 30 年里,牛奶已经不再是三餐的标准饮料,所有年龄段的人都越发喜欢喝软饮料、果汁和其他饮料。如果没有足够的牛奶摄入,儿童几乎不可能从饮食中获得所需的钙。而儿童成长需要大量的钙摄入。"

研究人员表示钙只在人体 20 岁之前对骨骼生长有作用。此后,无论你服用多少钙,骨质都不会增加,但骨质流失的缓慢过程很快就开始了。对成年人而言,钙最好的作用是减缓骨质流失。因此,如今缺钙的儿童随着年龄的增长患骨质疏松症的风险要大得多,甚至会出现更多的骨折现象。

**课文 B**

### 骨折

当外力作用于骨骼时,骨骼便有断裂的风险。如果骨骼不能承受这些外力,就会发生骨折。骨折发生时,骨骼将失去完整性,骨结构将被破坏。

根据骨折发生部位和外观等特点,骨折可分为许多种类。如果骨折处皮肤没有破裂,称为闭合性骨折。开放性骨折时,皮肤破裂,暴露骨头,伤口更易于感染。如果骨骼全部折断,被称为完全骨折;如果是部分折断则被称为不完全骨折(或青枝骨折)。青枝骨折在儿童中更为常见。若骨骼承受长期重复活动带来的压力而破裂,称为压力性骨折。根据骨折线的方向不同,分为横形骨折、斜形骨折、螺旋形骨折。如果骨折形成多个碎块,则称为粉碎性骨折。事实上,骨折可能为单一类型,也可能同时存在多种类型骨折。

一般来说,骨折会导致疼痛、肿胀,有时会因内出血而出现淤伤。患者不能承受重力或压力,移动时会产生剧烈疼痛。骨折周围的软组织也可能受伤。若患处脉搏丧失,骨折周围或其以下部位可能会出现麻木或瘫痪。

可通过对患处进行检查和 X 线片检查来确诊骨折。然而,某些类型的骨折在 X 线片上很难看到。在这种情况下,医生可能会要求患者进行其他诊断性影像学检查,如计算机断层扫描、磁共振成像或骨骼扫描。开放性骨折需要额外的实验室检查以确定是否存在失血和感染。

在野外对手臂、腿、手和足骨折的初步治疗包括肢体原位夹板固定、抬高患肢和局部冰敷。固定患处对初始疼痛控制非常有帮助。对于颈部和背部损伤,急救人员或护理人员可将伤者放置在长形木板上并戴上颈托,以保护脊髓免受潜在损伤。

骨折手术在很大程度上取决于骨折类型和骨折部位。外科医生对骨折进行处理,使骨骼位置复原,然后用石膏固定。有时,骨折处需要植入金属来固定。根据骨折情况的不同,有些金属是永久放入不再取出,有些只是暂时安放,在完全愈合一段时间后再通过手术取出。

# Unit 9　The Oral Cavity

**课文 A**

### 牙龈炎与牙周疾病

嘴巴的第一部分被称为口腔。沿着口腔边的前面到侧边是两个包含牙齿的拱形。口腔还包括舌头、硬腭、软腭、小舌和牙龈。这个整体结构也被称为嘴巴。口腔内部结构使我们能够品尝和咀嚼食物、吞咽食物、喝饮料，并且能够控制从喉咙里出来的空气，使我们能说话。

与口腔有关的常见问题包括口臭、蛀牙、牙龈疾病、口腔癌以及口腔溃疡。为了预防这些问题，人们可以每天刷牙两次，每天使用牙线，每年至少做一次口腔癌检查，避免吸烟，吃健康的食物或者约每两个月更换一次牙刷。

牙龈炎，或者称牙龈炎症，通常发生在牙周炎或牙龈疾病之前。在牙龈炎的早期，牙菌斑中的细菌积聚导致牙龈发炎，并且刷牙的时候容易出血。虽然牙龈可能受到刺激，但是牙齿依然牢牢地长在牙槽中。在这个阶段没有发生不可逆的骨骼或者其他组织损伤。

如果牙龈炎得不到治疗，就会导致牙周炎。患有牙周炎的人，牙龈和骨头的内层会从牙齿上脱落，形成洞。牙齿和牙龈之间的这些小空洞会残留一些牙齿碎片，并且可能感染。当牙菌斑在牙龈线以下扩散和生长时，人体的免疫系统会开始对抗细菌。

这时牙菌斑中的细菌产生的毒素，以及人体抵抗感染的"好"酶，开始破坏固定牙齿的骨骼和结缔组织。随着病情的加剧，牙槽变深，更多的牙龈组织和骨骼被破坏。当这种情况发生时，牙齿不再固定在原有的位置，它们开始松动，出现脱落。并且牙龈看起来是苍白的，而不是健康的粉红色。牙龈疾病是成年人牙齿脱落的主要原因。

人们可以通过每天刷牙、用牙线清洁牙齿、戒除不良的口腔习惯（如吸烟）来预防牙龈炎和牙周炎。

**课文 B**

### 口腔癌在年轻人中日益流行

现在越来越多的年轻人患上了口腔癌，这种现象向人们发起了预警。

过去一度认为那些年纪大的人更容易患口腔癌，但从目前情况来看，该病在年轻人和女性中正呈现出与日俱增的发展趋势。

年轻人过度饮酒和吸烟可能是导致口腔癌在该群体中发病率上升的两个"帮凶"。

英国口腔卫生基金会最近向年轻人发出警告说，如果想要遏制口腔癌不断攀升的发病率，那么他们就必须立即开始对自己的口腔进行定期检查。

在过去 10 年中，患口腔癌的女性与男性的比例增加了三分之一，尽管男性患口腔癌的可能性仍然是过去的两倍。

口腔癌的发病部位包括嘴唇、舌头、面颊和喉咙。

在英国，每年有 4300 人被确诊患口腔癌，而每年死于该病的人数则为 1700 人。

口腔癌常见的原因是吸烟和饮酒过量，两者都有的人患这种疾病的概率是不吸烟的人的 30 倍。

饮食不良也与口腔癌有关。

但英国口腔卫生基金会认为，在年轻人中，约 25％ 的口腔癌病例没有涉及这些常见的危险因素。英国口腔卫生基金会认为，这意味着即使人们有着健康的生活方式，但知道口腔癌可能的症状也是至关重要的。

# Unit 10　The Reproductive System

**课文 A**

### 生殖系统概论

生殖系统是一组内部器官和外部器官的总称，在男性和女性中作用均是生育。由于生殖系统在物种生存中的重要作用，许多科学家认为生殖系统是整个身体中最重要的系统。

男性生殖系统由两个主要部分组成：产生精子的睾丸和阴茎。男性的阴茎和尿道既属于泌尿系统也属于生殖系统。睾丸位于一个被称为阴囊的外囊中，它们的温度通常比体温略低，有利于精子的产生。

女性生殖系统的主要内部器官包括阴道、子宫和卵巢。阴道和子宫是精液的容器,卵巢可以产生卵子。阴道通过过子宫颈与子宫相连,而输卵管连接子宫和卵巢。随着激素水平的变化,一个卵子或多个卵子会在排卵期间被释放进入输卵管。如果没有受精,这个卵子会随月经而消失。

受精就是精子进入输卵管并进入卵子的过程。受精通常发生在输卵管,也可能发生在子宫。当受精卵植入子宫内膜,胚胎开始形成(胚胎形成),然后胎儿开始形成。当胎儿发育成熟到足以在子宫外存活时,子宫颈扩张,子宫收缩推动其通过产道分娩。

课文 B

### 子宫内膜异位症

子宫内膜异位症是指子宫内膜细胞的异常生长。子宫内膜细胞每月都会在月经过程中脱落。这些细胞位于下腹部区域如输卵管和卵巢。然而,与子宫细胞不同的是,这些异常生长的细胞没有通道可以离开身体,所以停留在原地持续循环。在月经期间,正常的子宫内膜会脱落并从阴道排出,但植入的组织无法排出体外。结果就是内出血,出现炎症和瘢痕。这种瘢痕的严重后果之一就是不孕。这些细胞生长通常不是恶性的也不会癌变,但会破裂并扩散到新的区域。Redwine 博士描述了子宫内膜异位症的进行性病变:"首先表现为透明的小水疱,然后变成红色,在 7～10 年内发展为黑色。水疱在 4～10 年变成蓝色圆顶囊肿。平均 21.5 岁时可见明显病变,31.9 岁时可见黑色瘢痕。随着年龄的增长,从透明到红色到黑色的发展过程证实,如果不治疗疾病就会不断发展。在 47%～64% 的女性中,这种疾病不经治疗就会持续发展。"

研究人员正在研究用血液化验辅助检查子宫内膜异位症的症状。CA-125 是一种在中度或重度子宫内膜异位症中水平会升高的盆腔器官中的细胞蛋白。超声设备在诊断进行性子宫内膜异位症的大囊肿和其他特征时是必不可少的。正确使用腹腔镜检查通常能 100% 准确诊断子宫内膜异位症。不使用腹腔镜,通常不能确诊子宫内膜异位症。腹腔镜检查可显示肿瘤的位置、范围和大小。子宫内膜异位症的病因是个谜。目前还不清楚为什么有些女性会患上这种疾病,而另一些人看起来非常健康。其中血流逆行理论认为月经期间血流沿输卵管逆行会导致子宫内膜异位症。子宫内膜异位症在其母亲怀孕期间接受过 DES 激素治疗的女性和月经疼痛的女性中更为普遍。流传最广泛的理论认为,子宫内膜异位症是子宫内膜碎片附着在附近的盆腔结构后生长导致的。子宫内膜细胞在月经期中所有女性的腹膜液中都很常见。有人认为子宫内膜异位症会在所有女性中发生,事实并非如此。月经异常、大出血或月经期频繁、周期短、青春期发育早的女性更容易患子宫内膜异位症。另一种理论指出,激素问题致使这种组织在子宫内膜异位症女性体内生长。

子宫内膜异位症根据受累部位分为四个阶段。1 期,或轻度疾病:浅表和薄膜状粘连。2 期,或轻度疾病:浅表和深部子宫内膜异位,薄膜状粘连。3 期,或中度疾病:浅表和深部子宫内膜异位,薄膜状和致密性粘连。4 期,或严重疾病:浅表和深部子宫内膜异位,致密性粘连。尽管这些阶段看起来很相似,但还是可以根据病变区域的大小和数量进行诊断。这些症状似乎有助于确保正确的诊断,但除了子宫内膜异位症外,其他原因也可引起这些不适。还有一点很重要,注意并非所有患有这种疾病的女性都有症状,即使在疾病 4 期。尽管有些子宫内膜异位症女性没有症状,但疼痛在很多子宫内膜异位症病例中是个重要指标。据报道,疼痛在某种程度上干扰了日常生活的各个方面。78% 的人会干扰睡眠,这一发现很重要,因为疲劳会加速疼痛的严重程度。报道显示 100% 的人会在月经前 1～2 天有疼痛;71% 的人月经中期有疼痛;47% 的人其余时间也有疼痛;40% 的人全程疼痛;7% 的人无规律间歇性疼痛。疼痛一旦发生,81% 的人认为疼痛是进行性的。在描述疼痛时的情绪和感受时,84% 的人感到沮丧,75% 的人易怒,63% 的人经历过情绪波动,54% 的人感到焦虑,53% 的人愤怒,51% 的人消极,43% 的人无助,35% 的人恐惧无力,32% 的人担心,31% 的人没有安全感,19% 的人感到没有希望。尽管激素疗法在缓解症状方面可能有一定效果,但会产生令人不快的副作用。

# Appendix D   Keys to the Exercises

**Unit 1**

**Task 1**

1. E   2. A   3. B   4. C   5. D

**Task 2**

(1)(2)(4)(3)

**Task 3**

1. fever   2. sore throat   3. runny nose   4. headache   5. blood test

**Task 4**

1. upper   2. take aspirin   3. three times

**Task 5**

1. circulation   2. delivery   3. nutrition   4. approximate   5. systematically
6. prevalence   7. unhealthy   8. Urbanization   9. industrial   10. preventive

**Task 6**

1. C   2. B   3. C   4. B   5. D

**Task 7**

4,2,3,1

**Task 8**

1. g   2. f   3. h   4. i   5. c   6. j   7. d   8. b   9. e   10. a

**Task 9**

1. A   2. B   3. C   4. D   5. A   6. B   7. C   8. D   9. A   10. B

**Task 10**

1. D   2. D   3. C   4. C   5. A   6. B   7. D   8. A   9. C   10. B

**Unit 2**

**Task 1**

1. B   2. D   3. A   4. E   5. C

**Task 2**

(5)(8)(1)(7)(3)(4)(2)(6)

**Task 3**

1. kidney function   2. liver function   3. biopsy   4. painful   5. swollen

**Task 4**

1. painkiller   2. kidney function   3. Chinese traditional herbs

**Task 5**

1. glycerol   2. digestive   3. salivary   4. carbohydrates   5. pancreatic
6. proteins   7. esophageal   8. abdomen   9. absorbing   10. alimentary

*Note*

153

**Task 6**

1. D  2. D  3. A  4. C  5. B

**Task 7**

2,4,3,1

**Task 8**

1. f  2. h  3. g  4. c  5. i  6. j  7. e  8. b  9. d  10. a

**Task 9**

1. B  2. D  3. C  4. D  5. A  6. C  7. D  8. C  9. B  10. D

**Task 10**

1. A  2. C  3. A  4. B  5. B  6. D  7. C  8. D  9. B  10. C


**Unit 3**

**Task 1**

1. E  2. C  3. D  4. A  5. B

**Task 2**

(4)(1)(2)(3)

**Task 3**

1. GI department  2. admitting  3. Nov. 15<sup>th</sup>  4. stools  5. positive

**Task 4**

1. pressure  2. good  3. palpitations

**Task 5**

1. bacteria  2. infectious  3. bronchitis  4. allergy  5. complication
6. chronic  7. recur  8. contagiousness  9. drainage  10. viruses

**Task 6**

1. C  2. D  3. D  4. A  5. B

**Task 7**

3,1,5,2,6,4

**Task 8**

1. g  2. e  3. f  4. h  5. b  6. a  7. i  8. d  9. j  10. c

**Task 9**

1. C  2. B  3. A  4. D  5. D  6. B  7. A  8. C  9. A  10. C

**Task 10**

1. D  2. A  3. B  4. C  5. B  6. A  7. C  8. A  9. C  10. C


**Unit 4**

**Task 1**

1. B  2. C  3. D  4. E  5. A

**Task 2**

(2)(3)(4)(5)(6)(1)

**Task 3**

1. Blood pressure, pulse rate and breathing rate  2. fluids  3. chart

**Task 4**

1. secondary line  2. nutrients  3. sticky, blockage

*Note*

**Task 5**

1. center  2. nervous  3. containing  4. accident  5. neurologist
6. incredibly  7. unhealthy  8. reproductive  9. removal  10. preventive

**Task 6**

1. D  2. C  3. D  4. A  5. A

**Task 7**

1,4,3,2

**Task 8**

1. i  2. j  3. g  4. h  5. e  6. f  7. d  8. c  9. b  10. a

**Task 9**

1. A  2. D  3. C  4. B  5. C  6. A  7. B  8. A  9. D  10. A

**Task 10**

1. C  2. B  3. D  4. C  5. A  6. D  7. A  8. B  9. C  10. D

**Unit 5**

**Task 1**

1. C  2. A  3. D  4. E  5. B

**Task 2**

1. roller clamp  2. IV solution bag  3. IV stand  4. catheter

**Task 3**

1. headache  2. dizzy  3. prescribed  4. lower  5. instructions

**Task 4**

1. melt  2. absorbing, salt  3. dietary fiber

**Task 5**

1. functional  2. regulation  3. grow  4. reproduction  5. Nerves
6. message  7. secretion  8. extensively  9. infectious  10. location

**Task 6**

1. D  2. B  3. C  4. A  5. B

**Task 7**

3,1,2

**Task 8**

1. c  2. f  3. h  4. e  5. a  6. j  7. d  8. i  9. g  10. b

**Task 9**

1. B  2. B  3. C  4. D  5. A  6. C  7. A  8. B  9. D  10. A

**Task 10**

1. A  2. C  3. D  4. A  5. B  6. C  7. A  8. C  9. B  10. D

**Midterm Review**

Ⅰ **Listening**

1. B  2. D  3. H  4. G  5. E  6. A  7. B  8. B  9. A  10. A
11. 36 ℃  12. 64  13. 110/70 mmHg  14. 18  15. 98%  16. 60 kg

Ⅱ **Reading and Writing**

**Part 1**

1. B  2. A  3. C  4. C  5. B  6. A  7. B  8. C  9. C  10. A

**Part 2**

1. C   2. B   3. A   4. B   5. C   6. B   7. B   8. A   9. B   10. A

**Part 3**

1. wash   2. check   3. prime   4. Set   5. connect   6. start   7. sign   8. write up

**Part 4**

The patient was called Tom Smith. He was 15 years old. He was admitted to hospital because of high fever, dry cough and no appetite on May 15th, 2020. He was diagnosed as pneumonia and placed on erythromycin to dephlogisticate by attending physician Dr. John. After 10 days' treatment, the patient improved, showing general state of health. And the patient had good appetite. The patient was discharged in stable condition. At last, he was diagnosed as pneumonia and Dr. John told the patient that no medication needed after discharge. The patient should follow up with Dr. John in one week.

**Unit 6**

**Task 1**

1. B   2. E   3. A   4. C   5. D

**Task 2**

1. commode chair   2. shower chair   3. walking frame

4. walking stick   5. crutches   6. wheelchair

**Task 3**

1. surgery   2. risks   3. anesthesia   4. bleeding   5. standard   6. low-residue   7. fluids

**Task 4**

1. around 8:00 pm   2. bowel movement   3. stomach

**Task 5**

1. genetic   2. affected   3. providers   4. clinics   5. screening

6. treatment   7. disability   8. sufferings   9. diagnosed   10. Potential

**Task 6**

1. C   2. B   3. A   4. C   5. B

**Task 7**

1, 5, 2, 4, 3, 6, 7

**Task 8**

1. i   2. g   3. f   4. a   5. c   6. e   7. b   8. j   9. d   10. h

**Task 9**

1. C   2. B   3. B   4. D   5. A   6. B   7. D   8. C   9. A   10. D

**Task 10**

1. B   2. D   3. A   4. C   5. B   6. D   7. A   8. C   9. B   10. D

**Unit 7**

**Task 1**

1. A   2. B   3. E   4. C   5. D

**Task 2**

(3) (1) (5) (2) (6) (4)

**Task 3**

1. admitted   2. recovered   3. vital   4. normal   5. blood circulation

**Task 4**

1. wash, clean, gloves   2. cover, stoma   3. close

**Task 5**

1. sensation   2. urinary   3. filters   4. urethritis   5. cystitis

6. discomfort   7. promptly   8. painful   9. bacterium   10. infection

**Task 6**

1. C   2. D   3. D   4. A   5. B

**Task 7**

1,3,2,4,5

**Task 8**

1. f   2. e   3. h   4. g   5. b   6. a   7. d   8. c

**Task 9**

1. D   2. B   3. A   4. C   5. B   6. D   7. C   8. D   9. C   10. C

**Task 10**

1. C   2. D   3. B   4. A   5. C   6. A   7. B   8. D   9. C   10. B


**Unit 8**

**Task 1**

1. B   2. A   3. C   4. E   5. D

**Task 2**

(5) (2) (3) (1) (4) (6)

**Task 3**

1. took some medicine   2. ordered   3. enema   4. handle

**Task 4**

1. identification   2. on her left side   3. 5-10

**Task 5**

1. pediatrician   2. orthopedics   3. surgeon   4. fractured   5. essentially

6. deficient   7. adequately   8. virtually   9. critically   10. osteoporosis

**Task 6**

1. D   2. A   3. C   4. C   5. B

**Task 7**

1,3,2,4,6,5

**Task 8**

1. e   2. f   3. g   4. i   5. j   6. a   7. b   8. c   9. d   10. h

**Task 9**

1. C   2. B   3. C   4. B   5. A   6. A   7. B   8. B   9. A   10. C

**Task 10**

1. A   2. B   3. C   4. D   5. D   6. C   7. B   8. A   9. A   10. B


**Unit 9**

**Task 1**

1. B   2. D   3. A   4. C   5. E

**Task 2**

(4) (5) (6) (2) (1) (3)

*Note*

157

**Task 3**

1. diabetes   2. educate you   3. insulin   4. prescribed   5. regular

**Task 4**

1. before her meal   2. disposable and easy   3. food

**Task 5**

1. manipulating   2. abstain   3. decay   4. immunize   5. irritate

6. swallowing   7. screened   8. chew   9. infect   10. inflamed

**Task 6**

1. D   2. C   3. B   4. A   5. D

**Task 7**

1, 4, 3, 2

**Task 8**

1,d;   2,c;   3,e;   4,j;   5,h;   6,a;   7,b;   8,i;   9,g;   10,f;

**Task 9**

1. D   2. B   3. C   4. B   5. C   6. A   7. C   8. A   9. C   10. C

**Task 10**

1. A   2. B   3. C   4. D   5. D   6. C   7. B   8. A   9. B   10. B


**Unit 10**

**Task 1**

1. C   2. D   3. E   4. B   5. A

**Task 2**

(2) (3) (1)

**Task 3**

1. urine   2. bathroom   3. infection   4. antibiotics   5. skin test

**Task 4**

1. identification bracelet   2. relax   3. call bell

**Task 5**

1. urinary   2. contraction   3. uterus   4. survived   5. reproductive

6. hormonal   7. fertilization   8. collection   9. slightly   10. ovum

**Task 6**

1. B   2. D   3. A   4. A   5. C

**Task 7**

1,3,4,2,6,5

**Task 8**

1. h   2. a   3. i   4. b   5. j   6. d   7. e   8. f   9. g   10. c

**Task 9**

1. D   2. A   3. C   4. B   5. B   6. A   7. C   8. B   9. D   10. B

**Task 10**

1. C   2. D   3. A   4. C   5. B   6. A   7. C   8. D   9. C   10. A


**Final Review**

Ⅰ **Listening**

1. B   2. E   3. A   4. C   5. F

6. A  7. A  8. B  9. B  10. A

11. A  12. B  13. C  14. B  15. B

## II Reading and Writing

**Part 1**

1. check  2. prime  3. set  4. connect  5. start  6. sign  7. write up

**Part 2**

1. F  2. A  3. C  4. E  5. D

**Part 3**

1. A  2. C  3. B  4. A  5. B  6. B  7. A  8. B  9. A  10. C

**Part 4**

Hospice Care

Recently, when it comes to the question "what do the patients who are at the end of their lives need", hospice care or palliative care is always advocated. So there are a growing number of hospitals are offering the hospice care.

With the fast yet steady economic and social development, people begin to pay more attention to the terminally ill patients. Because we can't cure all the diseases but medical workers can make those patients feel more comfortable before they leave the world.

As what we can see, it really doesn't matter whether we can make the patients recovered from the illness, but the hospice care they get at the end of their lives. First the patients can become more comfortable. What's more, the patients are treated with dignity and respect through hospice care. At last, the patients' family can get their burden lessened because they don't need to spend too much money on medications.

*Note*